PROBABILITY MODELS AND CANCER

PROBABILITY MODELS AND CANCER

Proceedings of an Interdisciplinary Cancer Study Conference
Berkeley, July 1981

edited by

Lucien LE CAM

and

Jerzy NEYMAN †

Department of Statistics
Statistical Laboratory
University of California
Berkeley, CA, U.S.A.

RC 267
I 5256
1981

1982

NORTH-HOLLAND PUBLISHING COMPANY – AMSTERDAM • NEW YORK • OXFORD

© North-Holland Publishing Company, 1982

All rights reserved. No part of this publication may be reproduced, stored in a retrieval system, or transmitted in any form or by any means, electronic, mechanical, photocopying, recording or otherwise, without the prior permission of the copyright owner.

ISBN: 0 444 86514 4

Publishers:
NORTH-HOLLAND PUBLISHING COMPANY
AMSTERDAM • NEW YORK • OXFORD

Sole Distributors for the U.S.A. and Canada:
ELSEVIER SCIENCE PUBLISHING COMPANY, INC.
52 VANDERBILT AVENUE, NEW YORK, N.Y. 10017

Library of Congress Cataloging in Publication Data

Interdisciplinary Cancer Study Conference (1981 :
   University of California)
   Probability models and cancer.

   Papers from a conference held July 1981.
   1. Cancer--Research--Statistical methods--Congresses.
2. Cancer--Mathematical models--Congresses. 3. Prob-
abilities--Congresses. I. Le Cam, Lucien M. (Lucien
Marie), 1924-   . II. Neyman, Jerzy, 1894-   .
III. Title. [DNLM: 1. Medical oncology--Congresses.
2. Models, Biological--Congresses. QZ 200 I599p 1981]
RC267.I5256 1981   616.99'4'0072   82-18770
ISBN 0-444-86514-4 (U.S.)

PRINTED IN THE NETHERLANDS

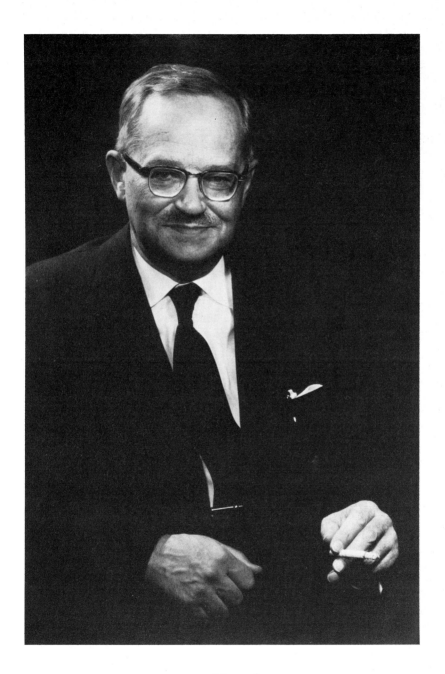

Jerzy Neyman

Jerzy Neyman

1894-1981

In the late Spring 1981, Professor Neyman approached us with the idea that there should be an interdisciplinary conference for an exchange of ideas between statisticians and biologists working on Cancer. Furthermore, he wanted that conference to take place forthwith, or at the latest in early July. In the short time available, organization of such a meeting appeared difficult to impossible, but Neyman went at it with his usual energy and enthusiasm and there was a conference.

Neyman is well known for his fundamental contributions to the very foundations of the science of Statistics. He is also well known for his contributions to applications of Statistics to various domains, extending from Astronomy to Weather Modifications. His involvement in the subject of Cancer dates back to the late fifties when he spent three months at N.I.H. in Bethesda. This involvement led to over 20 years of research activity on the subject. At first Neyman was interested in the design of experiments that would distinguish between the one stage and multiple stage theories of carcinogenesis. He arranged for such experiments to be performed. Some of the history is recounted in his own paper in the present volume. Later on Neyman became interested in the action of radiation on organisms and on single cells. His efforts with P. S. Puri, led to elaboration of complex stochastic models and of a search for data that would either corroborate such models or show their deficiencies. The search for data was at first fruitless. However we learned, from Dr. Hackett and Dr. Ainsworth, that Dr. Yang was developing precisely such experimental data in a laboratory within walking distance from our own offices. At this point Neyman determined that it was imperative that we meet and exchange ideas with at least some of the people working on carcinogenesis, mutagenesis and related subjects. Hence the conference whose Proceedings are in the present volume.

As already mentioned, the organizational task appeared difficult to impossible. In order to insure some impact on other workers in the field, Proceedings should be prepared and published. There was no time to secure Federal funds and our University dragged its administrative feet. Neyman proceeded along, with vigor, and made from his personal funds a grant to cover all expenses. The conference turned out to be an unqualified success. However shortly thereafter, Neyman was stricken and, after a short hospitalization, passed away. As was characteristic of him, he worked in the hospital to the very last hour before his demise.

He has left us with a monumental scientific heritage. His death marks the end of a remarkable era in the subject of statistics itself, an era marked by the names of Neyman, Pearson, Fisher, and Wald, whose contributions constitute the very basis of our science and methodology. But Neyman's legacy extends far beyond ordinary statistical methodology. He always insisted on the construction of stochastic models of natural phenomena, based on the available knowledge in the field. This meant delving into the subject itself and coming up with formulas with at least some semblance of relation to reality. In all of this he was great and was an inspiration to many.

We regret that he did not live to see the publication of the present Proceedings. However we would like, fondly and respectfully, to dedicate them to his memory.

Introduction

This is a collection of papers presented at a short Cancer Study Conference organized by J. Neyman and L. Le Cam in July 1981. The purpose of the conference was to improve communication between statisticians and scientists studying cancer in the laboratory, or in real life. The former group is often asked for advice on particular matters. Some of its members also have a genuine interest in the subject itself. They can propose mathematical models that should aid in understanding what happens in the laboratory and in life. However, some knowledge of the facts and some understanding of their relationships are indispensable, if the models are to be at all realistic. The conference itself provided a forum for interaction between several groups. It is our hope that the papers collected here will further such interest and cooperation.

The papers on the "substance" of the subject were kindly presented by their authors at a level accessible to statisticians. They cover many different aspects of the field. Dr. Hackett tells us about cell cultures maintained in her laboratory at the Peralta Cancer Research Institute. They have many uses in studying the structure of normal and abnormal cells and their reactions to various stimuli. It appears that tumors of the same generic name differ, but that even within a given tumor there is a surprisingly large variability that should be taken into account in the design of a drug cocktail appropriate to the chemotherapy of that tumor.

The paper by V. S. Byers *et al.* deals with the curious properties of monoclonal antibodies directed against osteosarcoma tumors. They do not bind to normal cells, but do recognize a number of other tumors, including several carcinomas. They can, and will be, used as "magic bullets" that stick to abnormal cells and inject them with toxins. They are most valuable in studies of antigen expression in normal and transformed cells.

Every one of us lives in a sea of mutagens. Joyce McCann and Renae Magaw tell us about the statistical problems involved in calibrating the various tests for mutagenicity and in the development of a suitable scale for mutagenic potency.

The paper by J. Ainsworth is a short treatise on the mutagenic, carcinogenic and other deleterious properties of radiation. It covers much of the current knowledge on dose-rate, dose fractionation effects, and comparison of "biological efficiency" of various forms of radiation.

There are two other papers on the effects of radiation. It turns out that J. Neyman and P. S. Puri had proposed a mathematical model of the effect of radiation on isolated cells in culture. It happens also that Tracy Yang and his colleagues were finding out experimentally what occurs if one irradiates cells in culture. Whether the mathematics and the laboratory results fit together is not yet known, but shall be in a few months. The Neyman-Puri equations include a time variable absent in previous models, even deterministic ones. Special experiments may be needed to verify that time does indeed play a role of the kind implied by the equations.

A very interesting development in cancer studies has been the discovery that genes responsible for the damage done in cases of transformation by viruses may be some of our own genes, which perform useful functions under normal conditions but are made overeager by viral action or other stimuli. The story is told very briefly by H. Oppermann.

Professor H. Rubin reminds us that an organism is more than just a congregation of separate cells. In his challenging view, the organization of cells in a tissue is a most important aspect, often neglected in the literature. By forcing malignant cells to "organize" themselves in close proximity, he can make them forget their malignant dispositions for a few generations. The mathematical problem of formulating models in which such organization is accounted for appears formidable.

On mathematical models, we have presentations by Bühler, Bartoszyński, Clifford, Le Cam, and Puri (mentioned earlier). P. Clifford shows that very different mathematical models may well be indistinguishable, no matter how many observations are made. That creates real difficulties because, within the limits of non-identifiability, different models may suggest different predictions, policies, and therapies.

Neyman's paper deplores the fact that even with "serial sacrifices", lack of identifiability remains. Many important biological parameters cannot be estimated. He suggests the development of "non invasive" procedures to monitor the laboratory animals' health.

Although it was not planned that way, the papers by Bühler, Bartoszyński and Le Cam encountered a common theme: some of the most often used mathematical models of tumor growth or metastasis simply do not fit the observable facts.

Prehn's theory of carcinogenesis through clonal selection says that chemical carcinogens act, not by transforming cells, but by damaging normal cells more severely than some that already had undergone some transformation. Bühler shows that a model built on this assumption does not fit the facts.

The paper by Bartoszyński *et al.* and the paper by Le Cam point out that a very commonly used model, implicit in simplified form in much of the medical literature on tumor growth, just does not fit, and in fact is off by factors of 10^5. The two groups of authors differ strongly on the interpretation of the lack of fit and on how to fix it.

R. Bohrer considers a different problem: what statistical tests should be used if you are trying out various chemicals and their combinations for mutagenicity or carcinogenicity? The problem of optimal selection of the statistical procedures does not have a clear-cut answer.

E. L. Scott reports a series of detailed statistical analyses on the effect of ultraviolet irradiation in mice. The effects are complex, depending on the UV wave lengths, dose rates fractionation, etc. The human epidemiological studies on skin cancer do seem to bear out a possible extrapolation from mice to men.

We hope that the papers printed here will give the reader an inkling of present knowledge and spur him or her to try to improve the state of the art.

Publication of the papers was made possible by the services of North Holland Publishing Company. Preparation of the camera-ready copies involved many of our associates. Particular thanks are due to Monica Jackson, Richard Eskow, Marilyn Hill, and, for the technically difficult parts of the process, to Richard Haney.

I wish to extend thanks also to my students and colleagues who proofed manuscripts at various stages of the process. The responsibility for the flaws that remain are not theirs, but mine.

July 13, 1982

Contributors

E. John Ainsworth, Biophysics, Donner Laboratory, Berkeley, California
Robert W. Baldwin, Cancer Research Campaign Laboratories, Nottingham, England
J. Bartley, Peralta Cancer Research Institute, Oakland, California
Robert Bartoszyński, Mathematical Institute, Polish Academy of Sciences, Warsaw, Poland
Robert Bohrer, Mathematics, University of Illinois at Urbana, Illinois
Barry W. Brown, Anderson Memorial Hospital, Houston, Texas
Wolfgang Bühler, University of Mainz, W. Germany
Vera S. Byers, University of California, San Francisco and Veterans Administration Hospital, Martinez, California
Peter Clifford, Oxford University, Oxford, England
M. James Embleton, Cancer Research Campaign Laboratories, Nottingham, England
Adeline J. Hackett, Director, Peralta Cancer Research Institute, Oakland, California
Lucien Le Cam, Statistics, University of California, Berkeley, California
Norbert Lenz, University of Mainz, W. Germany
Alan S. Levin, University of California, San Francisco, California
Renae S. Magaw, Biochemistry, Lawrence Berkeley Laboratory, Berkeley, California
Joyce McCann, Biochemistry, Lawrence Berkeley Laboratory, Berkeley, California
Jerzy Neyman, Statistical Laboratory, University of California, Berkeley, California
Hermann Oppermann, Microbiology, University of California, San Francisco, California and Genentech Laboratories, San Francisco, California
Michael R. Price, Cancer Research Campaign Laboratories, Nottingham, England
Prem S. Puri, Statistics, Purdue University, West Lafayette, Indiana
Harry Rubin, Molecular Biology, University of California, Berkeley, California
Elizabeth L. Scott, Statistics, University of California, Berkeley, California
Helene S. Smith, Peralta Cancer Research Institute, Oakland, California

Martha R. Stampfer, Peralta Cancer Research Institute, Oakland, California

James R. Thompson, Anderson Memorial Hospital, Houston, Texas

Cornelius A. Tobias, Division of Biology and Medicine, Lawrence Berkeley Laboratory, Berkeley, California and Department of Biophysics and Medical Physics, University of California, Berkeley, California

Tracy C. H. Yang, Division of Biology and Medicine, Lawrence Berkeley Laboratory, Berkeley, California, and Department of Biophysics and Medical Physics, University of California, Berkeley, California

Opening Address

Jerzy Neyman
University of California, Berkeley

It gives me a great pleasure to open this conference intended to promote the interdisciplinary effort to study carcinogenesis.

I like to think of the present conference as the fourth of a sequence that started in 1977. The first conference of the sequence was organized by the Institute for Energy Analysis, Oak Ridge Associated Universities. It was a highly interdisciplinary conference. The participants included a substantial number of hosts, somehow connected with the institute, and about an equal number of statisticians from several centers in this country and a few from abroad. I attended this conference and have very pleasant memories. I learned at the Oak Ridge Conference many details of radiation related experiments on carcinogenesis that altered my perspective on the relative importance of certain statistical studies. The proceedings of the conference were published in 1978.

The second conference of the sequence occurred in 1979. It was also held at the Oak Ridge Institute for Energy Analysis, reflecting the conviction of the leading scholars there (Dr. Peter Groer) that the success of research in this particular domain depends on cross- fertilization.

As far as I know, the proceedings of the second Oak Ridge conference are not published, so that the ideas discussed do not reach research workers who did not attend the conference.

However, the two interdisciplinary conferences organized by "substantive" scholars at Oak Ridge inspired some statisticians. This inspiration is documented by a special session at the last summer's meeting of the Institute of Mathematical Statistics held on the Davis Campus of our

University. The session was labeled "Interdisciplinary Study of Carcinogenesis". The participants included Dr. J. M. Holland from Oak Ridge, whose ideas are very inspiring to me.

No attempt was made to publish the proceedings of the special session of Davis, which I consider as the third item of the sequence initiated in 1977 at Oak Ridge. Contrary to this, in organizing the present Cancer Study Conference a strong effort was made to have our Proceedings published. My hope is that they will appear *soon*!"

Table of Contents

Dedication	vii
Introduction	ix
List of contributors	xiii
Opening address	xv
1. Hackett, A. J., Stampfer, M. R., Bartley, J., and Smith, H. S., "*The Cellular Biology of Mammary Cancer: Potential Resource for Biostatisticians*".	1
2. Byers, V. S., Baldwin, R. W., Levin, A. S., Embleton, M. J., and Price, M. R., "*Development of Monoclonal Antibodies to Osteogenic Sarcoma; Potential Uses*".	15
3. Bühler, W. J., and Lenz, N., "*Chemical Carcinogenesis and Clonal Selection*".	35
4. Neyman, J., "*Avenue to Understanding the Mechanism of Radiation Effects: Extended Serial Sacrifice Experimental Methodology*".	45
5. Magaw, R., and McCann, J., "*Short-term Tests Used to Detect Mutagens and their Effects in Body Fluids*".	61
6. Clifford, P., "*Some General Comments on Nonidentifiability*".	81
7. Clifford, P., "*The Limits of Nonidentifiability in Time-dependent Compartment Models with Applications to Serial-sacrifice Experiments*".	85

8. Ainsworth, E.J., "*Radiation Carcinogenesis - Perspectives*".   99

9. Puri, P. S., "*A Hypothetical Stochastic Mechanism of Radiation Effects in Single Cells: Some Further Thoughts and Results*".   171

10. Yang, T. C., and Tobias, C. A., "*Studies on the Survival Frequencies of Irradiated Mammalian Cells With and Without Cancer Cell Morphology*".   189

11. Rubin, H., "*Some Remarks on Cancer as a State of Disorganization at the Cellular and Supracellular Levels*".   211

12. Scott, E. L., "*Response of Mice to Varying Times of UV Radiation*".   221

13. Oppermann, H., "*Viral and Cellular Oncogenes*".   245

14. Bartoszyński, R., Brown, B. W., and Thompson, J. R., "*Metastic and Systemic Factors in Neoplastic Progression*".   253

15. Le Cam, L., "*On Some Mathematical Models of Tumor Growth and Metastasis*". With discussion by Bartoszyński, R., Brown, B. W., and Thompson, J. R. Reply by Le Cam, L.   265

16. Bohrer, R., "*Optimal Multiple Decision Problems—Some Principles and Procedures Applicable in Cancer Drug Screening*".   287

The Cellular Biology of Mammary Cancer: Potential Resource for Biostatisticians

Hackett, A. J.

Stampfer, M. R.

Bartley, J., and

Smith, H. S.

University of California
Lawrence Berkeley Laboratory

Peralta Cancer Research Institute

1. The Cellular Biology of Mammary Cancer: Potential Resource for Biostatisticians

Mammary cancer is a highly variable disease and the basis for the variability is thought to be the cell of origin. Although most breast cancers are intraductal, they vary widely in morphological, behavioral and prognostic characteristics probably as a reflection of the stage in the differentiation process as well as the stage in malignant progression. In addition, the inductive basis for cancer may influence the nature of the disease.

There is epidemiological evidence that cancer in humans results from an interaction of multiple factors and that there is a reversible stage in the induction of cancer (1). While there are several multifactorial and multistage model systems of cancer induction in experimental animals that have provided information about these and other phenomena associated with carcinogenesis (2, 3), extrapolation from animal models to human cancer has been difficult. One difficulty in studies on the cellular biology of human cancer stems from the heterogeneity of the human population and the lack of experimental systems which can separate individual differences from the properties common to all humans. Recently developed technology for growth of epithelial cells in culture should provide us with the means to resolve at least part of that dilemma, (4, 5), and also test the validity of the animal model systems used in the study of cancer.

A human epithelial culture system would ideally fulfill several requirements: (a) epithelial cells must be successfully grown from *every* donor regardless of age, disease, state or background; (b) the system must permit the amplification of a small number of cells in the specimen to very large numbers in a very short time with minimal alteration from the original *in vivo* state; (c) the cells must be viable after storage in the frozen state. Our human mammary epithelial cell culture system meets these criteria.

At Peralta Cancer Research Institute we have developed the technology for growth in culture of human mammary epithelial cells from normal and malignant breast tissue (5). Techniques have been developed for cryopreservation as well as for rapid replication of epithelial cells to very large numbers, at low passage, without contamination with other cell types. Epithelial cells can be grown from nonmalignant and tumor tissue from a single donor, as well as from donors with different histopathological types of breast disease, different ages and backgrounds. Comparisons within and between groups can be made.

2. Culturing Human Mammary Epithelium

The procedures for growth of human mammary epithelial cells in culture have been published in detail (5). Briefly, the ductal-alveolar elements of the breast tissue are dissected free of fat and grossly minced to pieces 0.5 cm in size. The tissue mince is treated with a mixture of collagenase and hyaluronidase until the stromal matrix and basement membranes have been hydrolyzed, releasing clumps of epithelial cells, free of adherent stroma. The clumps are isolated by filtration and washed free of enzymes and single cells. These clumps or fragments of ducts and alveoli, termed organoids, can be cryopreserved. The organoids are suspended in preservation media (F-12-DME, 10% DMSO and 15% FCS) dispensed into ampoules, slow frozen, and stored in a liquid nitrogen freezer.

In the presence of an enriched growth medium, epithelial cells grow out from organoids plated on plastic surfaces. Normal mammary epithelial cells in primary and secondary culture grow with doubling times of 24 to 48 hours. More recently, growth has been extended to include rapid proliferation through fourth passage (at 1/10 dilution) by adding cholera toxin to the medium (6, 7). Most specimens (90%) derived from nonmalignant tissue, primary carcinomas and hypodermal metastases have been successfully cultured.

Certain experimental designs require single cell suspensions and clonal growth conditions. Such preparations can be readily obtained by dissociating primary outgrowths with trypsin to single cell suspensions suitable for clonal studies. Single cells, plated sparsely on fibroblast feeder layers in enriched medium, rapidly proliferate forming readily visible colonies with plating efficiencies ranging from 2 to 40% (7, 10). (Fig 1).

The cells in our cultures have been identified as epithelial in origin by morphology, ultrastructure, dome formation (5), presence of mammary specific milk fat globule antigen (6, 8), pattern of surface fibronectin (6, 9) and absence of endothelial markers (6). The identification of malignant cells is more difficult, but the fact that hypodermal metastases grow as well as primary carcinoma excludes the possibility that only nonmalignant cells present in the specimen are capable of growth in culture.

3. Cell Bank

The Institute has established a repository for human breast tissue specimens which provides a unique resource for investigators in fields of tumor cell biology, biostatistics and epidemiology. Since the specimen donors are local, follow-up information in addition to that already on file can be obtained.

Tables 1, 2, and 3 list the specimens in the Peralta Cancer Research Institute repository by age and pathology. Reduction mammoplasty

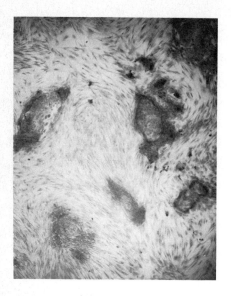 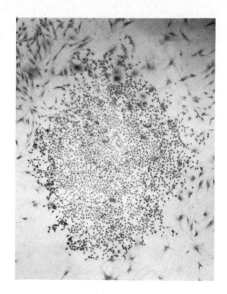

Fig. 1 Colony morphology of human mammary epithelial cell under clonal growth conditions.

A. Normal epithelial cell colonies from a reduction mammoplasty

B. Malignant epithelial cell colony from a metastatic breast carcinoma

specimens are shown in Table 1. A total of 57 are currently in the bank, 32 of which are under 30 years of age. The age of donors ranges from 16 to 68, providing specimens at puberty, as well as pre- and post-menopausal life stages. Age-matched specimens from donors with either normal or benign pathology are available.

Table 2 lists the tumor specimens in the bank. There are 61 tumor specimens, 24 of which are matched with tissue peripheral to the tumor. These specimens are particularly valuable since tissue peripheral to the tumor may provide experimental controls in the form of normal cells or cells at various stages in the progression to the malignant state. The collection provides controls not ordinarily available to scientists concerned with the heterogeneity in the human population. Although most of the tumors in the collection are intraductal carcinomas, a few of the less common

Table 1

Non-malignant Specimens in Peralta Cancer Research Institute Repository June 1981

Pathology	\-20	21-30	31-40	41-50	51-60	61-70	Total
Reduction Mammoplasties							
Normal	12	11	3	1	1	0	28
Fibrocystic Mastopathy	1	4	1	4	2	5	20
Mastectomies*	-	1	-	-	1	2	4
Fibroadenoma	1	3	1	2	0	0	7
	14	18	5	7	4	7	57

*Contralateral to tumor or subcutaneous

forms are represented, and more will be added to the collection as they become available.

Another facet of this repository is a unique collection of male breast specimens. One intraductal carcinoma and 6 benign specimens are available, two from donors under 20 years of age. These male breast cells will be useful in studies of cell to cell interaction where the sex marker chromosome can serve as an identifying marker.

Table 2

*Mastectomy Specimens in
Peralta Cancer Research Institute
Repository June 1981*

Type of Tissue	Age Unknown	21-30	31-40	41-50	51-60	61-70	71-80	Total
Comedo carcinoma (1 with peripheral)	-	-	-	2	-	-	-	2
Medullary carcinoma (with peripheral)	-	-	1	-	-	-	-	1
Lobular carcinoma (1 with peripheral)	-	-	-	2	2	-	-	4
Intraductal carcinoma								
Tumor only	2	2	1	6	6	4	6	27
Tumor & peripheral	-	-	1	6	4	5	6	22
Peripheral	3	1	2	3	0	1	2	12
	5	3	6	15	10	10	14	68

Table 3

Male Specimens in Peralta Cancer Research Institute Repository June 1981

Pathology	Age of Donor					
	20	21-30	31-40	41-50	51-60	Total
Gynecomasties	2	-	1	1	2	6
Intraductal Carcinoma	-	-	-	-	1	1
	2	-	1	1	3	7

4. Use of Human Cell System to Study Genetic Variability

A system for culturing human mammary epithelial cells has been developed. It is reliable, reproducible, easily manipulated and quantitative. It provides a system to study the following: heterogeneity in breast carcinomas at both the inter- and intra-tumor levels; comparison of tumor cell properties with those of normal cells from the same individual; and the effects of cell-cell interactions on the behavior of the various subpopulations in a tumor. Two on-going studies in our laboratory will be used to illustrate the flexibility of this culture system: (a) drug resistance; and (b) metabolism of benzo(a)pyrene.

5. Response to Adriamycin

Response to adriamycin in human mammary cell populations has been studied in our laboratory and is presented briefly here to illustrate the heterogeneity among breast carcinomas and the subpopulations within these tumors.

The clonal assay method is used to measure resistance to adriamycin. Primary cultures of human mammary tumor cells are trypsinized and the single cell suspension is seeded sparsely onto fibroblast feeder cells.

After allowing the epithelial cells to settle overnight, various concentrations of the drug are added for four hours, removed, the cell layer washed and additional feeder cells added in fresh growth medium. After 7 to 10 days incubation, the dishes are fixed, stained, and the colonies counted.

The quantitative data (colony numbers) can be plotted as percent survival on a linear scale to accentuate the differences among the various cell populations within each tumor (fig 2) or, on a logarithmic scale (fig 3) to emphasize the dose response of the most resistant fraction of the cell population. On a linear

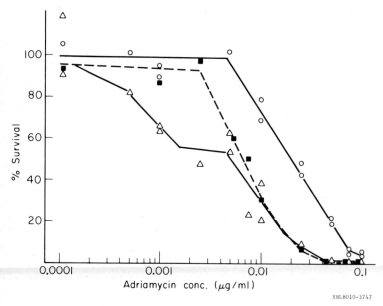

Fig. 2 Adriamycin toxicity of mammary carcinomas in second passage measured by clonal assay

-△- specimen 72T   --■-- specimen 173T   -0- specimen 82T

scale, one specimen, 72T, shows a biphasic response to adriamycin, with one component of the cell population more sensitive than another specimen (82T), and more resistant than a third specimen (173T). Fifteen-fold

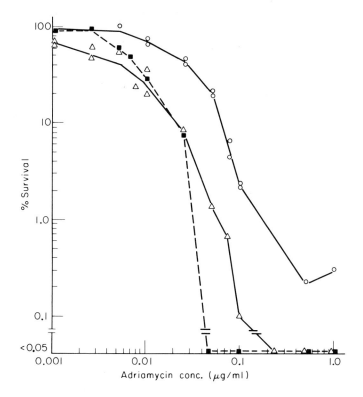

Fig. 3*   Adriamycin toxicity of mammary carcinomas in second passage measured by clonal assay

-Δ- 72T   --■-- 173T   -O- 82T

* Figures 2 and 3 are taken from reference 7 and reproduced with permission of the editors of Cancer Chemotherapy and Pharmacology.

differences in drug resistance are shown between these specimens, but differences as large as 65-fold have been obtained (Unpublished, Smith, et. al.). The characteristics of the most resistant fraction of the cell populations in the three specimens are emphasized by the log plot (fig 3). Specimen 72T is now shown to be more resistant than 173T, and 82T is shown to contain a very small cell component resistant to 1.0 μg/ml of the drug. Thus, the assay detects heterogeneity in response to adriamycin among breast carcinomas, and also detects subpopulations of cells within a single carcinoma.

Evaluation of the patient's tumor for drug sensitivity by this clonal assay has potential for basic studies on the mechanisms of drug resistance. However, if a high degree of positive association exists between the assay results and the patient's response, the assay could have great benefit to the patient by predicting the success of any proposed therapy and thus maximize therapeutic effectiveness.

6. Metabolism of BaP

The metabolism of a common chemical carcinogen, benzo(a)pyrene (BaP) by human mammary epithelial cells and the conditions which affect this metabolism provide another system to study genetic variability in humans. In contrast to studies with syngeneic animal models, wide individual variation may be expected when cells from various human donors are examined. Variation in metabolic patterns has been found with studies using organ cultures of human tissue; however, environmental exposure including nutritional intake in the 24 hours prior to excision of the tissue may influence these patterns. Such an environmental influence can be eliminated by culturing the cells for two to three passages prior to assay. It is possible that the organoid pools of breast epithelium may be able to detect the non-genetic variables in enzymatic patterns, while the cultured cells from the same pool may be used to determine the genetic component.

In experiments with human mammary epithelial cells exposed to 0.4 μM BaP, virtually all of the BaP was eliminated from the medium by 24 hrs incubation. There were differences between specimens in the pattern of metabolite products formed from the BaP. Specifically, the ratio of water soluble (non-toxic, non-mutagenic metabolites) versus organic soluble (including the putative mutagenic products) varied from 1.83 to 1 for three individual specimens (11).

When the DNA from epithelial cells from these three specimens was analyzed, the one exhibiting the lowest ratio of non-toxic to carcinogenic products had the highest amount of carcinogen modified DNA.

The DNA from cells grown out from nine specimens (7 normal, 2 tumor) was analyzed for the extent of binding of the putative carcinogenic product of BaP, the dial-epoxide, the mean number of these adducts was 1.82 for every 10^6 base pairs of DNA (Table 4).

Table 4

*Modification of DNA as a Consequence of BaP Metabolism
Human Mammary Epithelial Cells in Culture*

*BPDE Adducts/10^6 base pairs**

Donor No.	Normal cells derived from reduction mammoplasty specimens
H-3	1.68
H-48	0.84
H-51	0.59
H-97	1.61
H-123	2.18
H-183	3.62
H-184	1.90
	Tumor cells derived from mastectomy specimens
H-66T	1.40
H-157T	2.54

* Bases modified were 90% deoxyguanosine, 10% deoxycytidine.

The standard deviation was 0.91, a value in excess of the deviation found by replicate assays of cells grown out from a single donor. We interpret this deviation as an indication of inter individual variation. We do not as yet have sufficient data to determine the basis for this variation. Because the cells were in second to fourth passage, it is likely that the variation is due to genetic differences and will be reflected in measurable biochemical differences, e.g., enzymatic activities, membrane properties, DNA repair capability. In all cases, the same specific bases of DNA and in the same proportion were modified. This result suggests that the variation was in the extent of BaP metabolized and not at the stage of reacting with DNA.

Comparison of metabolism of BaP in epithelial cells with that of fibroblasts from the same donor showed a dramatic difference. At all concentrations tested, the epithelial cells form far more metabolites, both water-soluble and organic-solvent soluble than do the fibroblastic cells. These data show differences between cell types as well as individuals in the metabolism of the most ubiquitous carcinogen in our environment, and suggest that meaningful correlations with donor-genetic versus nutritional background, can be made. There may be metabolic patterns that segregate into groups, and these may correlate with various parameters such as lifestyle, cultural and genetic background. One possible result might be the identification of individuals at high risk for breast cancer.

7. Biological Variability in Human Breast Carcinomas

It has been noted that there is heterogeneity in the cellular populations that compose mouse mammary tumors (12, 13, 14). In that study, several cell lines obtained from a single tumor were shown to vary in the properties tested: antigenicity, morphology, karyotype, cloning efficiencies and tumorigenicity. Although a basic feature of human cancer is variability, there has not been a good human cell system available which could approach this problem.

Our human mammary cell culture system may provide the means to study tumor variability at the cellular level and extend our understanding of its basis. For example, variability in expression of drug resistance, antigens, morphology, cell-cell interactions, nutritional and hormonal requirements, may be easily quantitated using our highly efficient assay for clonal growth. These properties may be characterized for heterogeneity within a tumor cell population as well as among individual cells within a clonal derived colony. The data from the tumor specimens can be compared to that observed from non-malignant cell populations, permitting controlled studies on malignant progression.

Finally, the identification of donor characteristics that are associated with symptomatic disease and the expression of certain properties in culture are areas of research awaiting study, and now feasible with this reproducible assay system. Factors such as prior therapy, histological classification, level of risk for relapse should be examined for possible correlations with the characteristics of the donor's normal and tumor cells in culture. Computerization of accumulating data and subsequent analysis by biostatisticians, promises at least some clarification of the basis for the variability in human cancer.

8. Summary

Growth of human mammary epithelial cells in the mass culture system described has the potential to separate metabolic patterns that have a genetic basis from those due to environmental influences. Growth in the clonal mode where single cells are manipulated, permits study of heterogeneity within and between human mammary tumors at the cellular level. Both modes can provide the biostatistician and epidemiologist with the means to test old and new concepts on the genesis of human cancer.

9. References

1. Diamond, L., O'Brien, T. G. and Baird, W. M. in *Advances in Cancer Research 32*:1-63, 1980 - Academic Press, N. Y.
2. Boutwell, *Prog. Exp. Tumor Res. 4*:207-250, 1964.
3. Van Duuren, B. L. *Prog. Exp. Tumor Res. 11*:31-68, 1969.
4. Rheinwald, J. G. and Green, H. *Cell 6*:331-343, 1975 Yuspa, *Cancer Res. 40*:412-416, 1980.
5. Stampfer, M. R., R. Hallowes, A. J. Hackett. Growth of normal human mammary epithelial cells in culture. *In Vitro 16*:415-425, 1980.

6. Smith, H. S., Hackett, A. J., Riggs, J. L. et al. Properties of epithelial cells cultured from human carcinomas and nonmaglignant tissues. *J. Supramolecular Structure 11*:147-166, 1979.

7. Smith, H. S., Hackett, A. J., Lan, S. and Stampfer, M. R. Use of an efficient method for culturing human mammary epithelial cells to study adriamycin sensitivity. *Cancer Chemotherapy and Pharmacology*, in press, 1981.

8. Peterson, J. A., Bartholomew, J. C., Stampfer, M. R. and Ceriani, R. L. Quantitative changes in expression of human mammary epithelial (HME) antigens in breast cancer as measured by flow cytofluorimetry. *Cell Biol. 49*:1-14, 1981.

9. Stampfer, M. R., Vlodavsky, I., Smith, H. S. et al. Fibronectin production by human mammary cells in culture. *J. Natl. Cancer Inst. 67*:253-261.

10. Lan, S., Smith, H. S. and Stampfer, M. R. Clonal growth of normal and malignant human breast epithelia. *J. Surgical Oncology. 18*:#3, 1982.

11. Bartley, J., Bartholomew, J. C. and Stampfer, M. R. Metabolism of benzo(a)pyrene by human epithelial and fibroblastic cells: metabolite patterns and DNA adduct formation. *J. Supramolecular Structure*, in press.

12. Heppner, G. H., Shapiro, W. R. and Rankin J. K. G. B. Humphrey et al. (eds.) Cancer treatment and research; v. 2. 1. Tumors in children. 2. Neoplasms - In infancy and childhood - Period I. *Pediatric Oncology 1*:99-116, 1981.

13. Calabresi, P., Dexter, D. L. and Heppner, G. H. Clinical and pharmacological implications of cancer cell differentiation and heterogeneity. *Biochem. Pharmacol. 28*:1933-1941, 1979.

14. Dexter, D. L., Kawalski, H. M., Blazar, B. A. et al. Heterogeneity of tumor cells from a single mouse mammary tumor. *Cancer Res. 38*:3174-3181, 1978.

Monoclonal Antibodies: Their Use in the Diagnosis and Treatment of Cancer

*Vera S. Byers, Robert W. Baldwin, Alan S. Levin,
M. James Embleton, and Michael R. Price*

University of California San Francisco, Department of Dermatology and Cancer Research Campaign Laboratories, Nottingham England

1. Introduction

The field of tumor immunology had its beginnings in the 1930's with the demonstration that malignant tumors arising in one animal, when transferred to another preimmunized animal, are rejected. This suggested that tumor antigens existed on the surface of tumor cells, and these antigens could be specifically recognized by the immune system, resulting in tumor rejection. The field almost suffered a early demise with the discovery that histocompatibility antigens, and not tumor antigens, mediated this rejection. This discovery opened an important new field, that of transplantation immunology, but led to the conclusion that tumor antigens may not exist. In order to ascertain whether tumor antigens really do exist, it was necessary to wait for the production of inbred syngeneic animal strains to resolve this problem. Syngeneic animals are those that are genetically identical, and therefore tissues native to one animal are not rejected by the other. Using such animal strains, it was shown that chemically induced tumors could indeed be rejected by a preimmunized syngeneic host. (See the reviews by Byers and Baldwin, 1980, Woodruff, 1980.) During the next several decades, the field progressed dramatically, and the mechanism by which virally and chemically induced tumors are rejected on the basis of their tumor antigens were described. It was then suggested that the reason that cancers originate in a normal host might be due to a transient defect in their immune system.

The immune system is a complex network of cells and proteins which serve to protect the body from viruses, bacteria and fungi. The chief requirement for these agents to be destroyed is that they be recognized as foreign and non-self, and this is usually accomplished by the presence of a foreign chemical called an antigen. Thus, if the immune system is to be implicated in the death or shrinkage of tumors, it is necessary to demonstrate that they carry tumor associated antigens.

For example, virally induced tumors have a group of antigens which are found on all tumors induced by that virus. Chemically induced tumors have a series of unique antigens, some of which are shared on tumors produced by that chemical. All tumors carry a series of differentiation antigens, probably reflecting the fact that a tumor cell usually is the product of a maturational arrest, and appears far more dedifferentiated when compared to the normal cell in the organ from which it arose. Unfortunately, almost all of the studies on tumor immunology were done with chemically or virally induced tumors, since the time factor and low yield in finding spontaneously arising tumors is great. However, when these spontaneous tumors were ultimately tested it was found that only a few could be rejected by animals previously immunized with inactivated tumors (Hewitt, 1976). This leads to the conclusion that either spontaneous tumors in animals (rats were the source in this particular study) do not have tumor specific antigens, or that these antigens are not immunogenic. That is, these antigens can react in a specific immune response but cannot evoke an immune response *de novo*. To resolve this and many other problems in tumor immunology, many investigators are resorting to monoclonal antibodies.

The normal humoral immune response, even directed against a highly purified antigen, results in antibodies with a wide spectrum of activity and specificity. This leads to antisera which have affinities ranging from low to high, and more importantly, which will cross react with many closely related (but biologically different) antigens. This is a particular problem with human tumors, since such cells, when injected into animals, elicit the production of antibodies which are almost exclusively directed against the strong heterogeneic histocompatibility antigens. One way of dealing with this problem is by absorbing out the unwanted antibodies on affinity columns. If one attempts to absorb these antibodies out of the antiserum with normal tissues of the tumor donor, the weak antitumor antibodies usually are nonspecifically absorbed out as well. With the new techniques, monoclonal antibodies can be selected to have only one specificity, high affinity, and can be produced in large amounts by an immortal cell line.

2. Monoclonal Antibody Technique

The technique of immortalizing individual clones of antibody-secreting cells by fusing them with cultured cells of a mouse myeloma was developed by Köhler and Milstein (1975). In essence the technique depends upon the ability of two types of cells brought into close proximity to fuse and form heterokaryons. This tendency is vastly increased if the cells are exposed to certain agents such as UV-inactivated Sendai virus, lysolecithin, or polyethylene glycol. These heterokaryons can survive to produce their own progeny which inherit some of the characteristics of both parental cell types. The survival of hybrid progeny can be promoted by appropriate means of selection. In the case of antibody producing hybrids, one of the parental cell types consists of a lymphocyte population. These are usually lymphocytes from the spleen of an immunized animal, which contains actively dividing B cells. These B cells possess the genetic information for producing immunoglobulins with a definite specificity. However, they cannot survive indefinitely, since under normal circumstances they are "end-stage" cells, producing a certain quota of antibody and then dying. Therefore they are fused with a cancerous lymphocyte, a myeloma. This cell will proliferate indefinitely but lacks the capacity to produce a biologically meaningful immunoglobulin. The end result of the fusion is the production of hybrid cells which inherit the ability to produce highly specific antibodies and the ability for limitless division in culture.

In order to promote preferentially the growth of hybrid cells, there has to be selective pressure against unfused parental cells, or megakaryons formed by fusion between like cells. In the case of lymphocytes this presents no problem since they are incapable of unlimited proliferation and will rapidly die out when the fusion products are cultured. The unfused myeloma cells, however, require a more positive approach for their elimination, since they are selected for their ability for unlimited growth. In virtually all protocols this elimination is achieved by using mutant myelomas which lack an important enzyme such as thymidine kinase (or hypoxanthine-guanine phosophoribosyl transferase). These enzymes are part of the so-called "salvage pathways" present in normal cells. This allows normal cells to synthesize nucleic acids by an alternate pathway if they are cultured with chemicals which inhibit such synthesis by normal pathways. Thus the hybridomas which inherit these enzymes from their parental lymphocytes can grow in media containing the inhibitor aminopterin, while the unfused myelomas will die. Thus, progeny are selected which are composed only of fused cells.

When actively growing hybridomas appear, their supernatant medium needs testing for presence of antibody to the immunizing antigen. Many of the hybridomas secrete no antibody, and it is possible to eliminate these at an early stage by using radioimmunoassays for immunoglobulin in order to determine which supernatants actually contain antibody. These supernatants can then be tested against the relevant antigen, preferably including appropriate control targets (see below), to identify antibodies reacting against the component one is hoping to detect (Fig. 1). At this stage the chosen hybridoma(s) is cloned, either in soft agar or by limiting dilution, followed by further testing to select clones producing the desired monoclonal antibody. These hybridoma clones may then be propagated in culture (or sometimes in laboratory animals where appropriate) and so long as their chromosome complement remains stable, which is not always the case, they continue to secrete monoclonal antibodies, often in large amounts.

To date most of these hybridomas have been murine in origin, and most of the work in the field has been done with such hybridomas, either with murine tumors or with human tumors using murine antibodies. However, production of anti-measles antibody has been reported using entirely

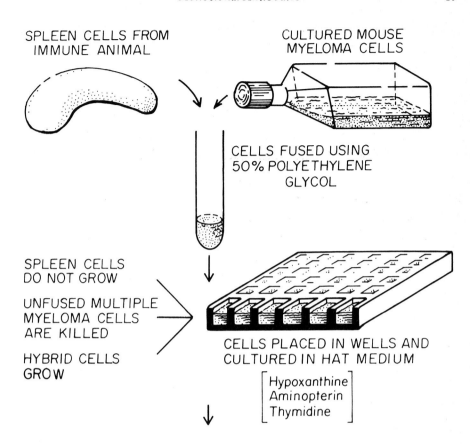

Figure 1

human hybridomas (Croce et al., 1980) and it is only a matter of time before the first reports of anti-tumor antibodies of human origin begin to appear.

3. Human Tumors; Osteogenic Sarcoma

In order to explore the possible uses of monoclonal antibodies to human tumors we chose initially to study osteogenic sarcoma in our laboratory. This choice was made partly because other studies had indicated that sarcomas may possess antigens which elicit a humoral antibody response in cancer patients (Morton and Malmgren, 1968; Bloom, 1972; Moore and Hughes, 1973; Byers *et al.*, 1975; Byers and Johnston, 1977; Rosenberg, 1980) and partly because cultured cell lines of osteogenic sarcomas, fibroblasts from the tumor-donors and serum samples from the autochthonous and allogeneic donors were available in the laboratory. This allowed the provision of adequate controls and a comparison between monoclonal antibodies produced *in vitro* and serum antibodies produced by the patient.

Murine monoclonal antibodies were made by immunizing BALB/c mice with cells of one of the osteogenic sarcoma lines, 791T, and fusing spleen cells from an immune mouse with the P3-NS1 myeloma line. Hybridoma supernatants were tested for reactivity against cultured tumor targets. Two of 48 hybridoma cultures resulting from a single fusion were found to react preferentially against the immunizing cell line, 791T, and a second (allogeneic) osteogenic sarcoma, 788T. Weaker reactivity by one of the hybridoma supernatants was obtained with a third osteogenic sarcoma (805T). The two hybridoma cultures (designated anti-791T/36 and anti-791T/48) were then cloned in soft agar and following cloning, 9 out of 12 clones were found to retain their specific reactivity against 791T (osteogenic sarcoma), but none reacted with either 791SK skin fibroblasts, lung fibroblasts or RAJI cells (Table 1). To test for purity and genetic stability, three of the nine positive clones were tested against an extensive panel of cells (Embleton et al., 1981) (Table 2). The reactivity of all three 791T/36 clones was identical, implying that only one antibody-producing clone was present in the original 791T/36 hybridoma. They were strongly positive

Table 1

Reactivity of Clones of Hybridoma 791T/36 Against 791T Osteogenic Sarcoma and Control Cell Lines

Test Supernatant	^{125}I cpm (±SD)[1] Bound to Target Cells:-			
	Osteogenic Sarcoma 791T[2]	Skin Fibroblasts 791SK[2]	Lung Fibroblasts 618 Lu	Burkitt Lymphoma Raji
HBSS + BSA[3]	278 ± 4	689 ± 15	396 ± 36	694 ± 31
P3NS1 spent medium	279 ± 50	410 ± 55	366 ± 6	485 ± 96
791T/36 Clone 1	12082 ± 402	326 ± 30	575 ± 52	719 ± 29
791T/36 Clone 2	14932 ± 598	380 ± 21	549 ± 22	522 ± 114
791T/36 Clone 3	16905 ± 261	404 ± 34	447 ± 6	444 ± 71
791T/36 Clone 4	16311 ± 322	316 ± 40	433 ± 33	473 ± 164
791T/36 Clone 5	10700 ± 388	339 ± 29	318 ± 8	591 ± 41
791T/36 Clone 6	13981 ± 371	361 ± 11	471 ± 9	632 ± 132
791T/36 Clone 7	921 ± 77	292 ± 14	307 ± 63	259 ± 36
791T/36 Clone 8	1174 ± 44	501 ± 51	369 ± 44	329 ± 36
791T/36 Clone 9	1858 ± 173	316 ± 16	455 ± 43	226 ± 24
791T/36 Clone 10	18333 ± 1236	334 ± 24	488 ± 19	229 ± 20
791T/36 Clone 11	18018 ± 63	657 ± 57	608 ± 118	276 ± 25
791T/36 Clone 12	11189 ± 497	425 ± 25	435 ± 57	323 ± 97

[1] Counts per minute ± standard deviation.
[2] 791T and 791SK were derived from the same patient.
[3] Hanks' balanced salt solution + 0.1% bovine serum albumin (washing medium).

Table 2

Reactivity of Certain 791T/36 Clones against Various Target Cells

		Binding ratio[1] of 791T/36 Clone:-		
Cell Line	Cell Type	Clone 3	Clone 4	Clone 10
791T[2]	Osteogenic sarcoma	22.84***	25.60***	22.84***
788T[3]	Osteogenic sarcoma	46.82***	53.13***	52.74***
845T	Osteogenic sarcoma	3.19*	5.58**	NT[5]
805T[4]	Osteogenic sarcoma	2.63	3.41*	2.99*
803T	Osteogenic sarcoma	1.45	1.45	NT
836T	Osteogenic sarcoma	0.78	0.73	0.82
706T	Osteogenic sarcoma	1.89	2.49	NT
781T	Osteogenic sarcoma	1.83	2.06	1.92
888T	Osteogenic sarcoma	1.08	1.13	1.12
792T	Osteogenic sarcoma	1.12	1.23	NT
791SK[2]	Skin fibroblasts	0.99	0.77	0.84
788SK[3]	Skin fibroblasts	0.90	NT	0.99
805SK[4]	Skin fibroblasts	1.41	2.05	1.46
181SK	Skin fibroblasts	2.14	2.18	2.10
836SK	Skin fibroblasts	1.31	1.29	NT
860[2]	Tumor-derived fibroblasts	1.39	NT	1.48
870[2]	Tumor-derived fibroblasts	1.09	1.04	0.95
618Lu	Lung fibroblasts	1.68	1.63	1.83
74BM	Foetal bone marrow	1.50	1.69	NT
-	Human erythrocytes	0.61-0.91	0.61-1.35	NT
-	Human mononuclear cells	0.61-1.24	0.70-2.00	0.63-1.28

Table 2 (con'd.)

Binding ratio[1] of 791T/36 Clone:-

Cell Line	Cell Type	Clone 3	Clone 4	Clone 10
(con'd.)				
HT29	Colon carcinoma	6.66**	7.10**	6.85**
HTC8	Colon carcinoma	1.61	2.52	1.89
HRT18	Colon carcinoma	1.21	1.02	1.10
734 B	Breast carcinoma	2.18	1.87	1.81
SK Br 3	Breast carcinoma	1.54	1.38	1.47
HS 578T	Breast carcinoma	1.22	1.76	1.32
MeWo	Melanoma	0.98	0.72	0.88
Mel 57	Melanoma	1.19	1.25	1.22
Mel 2a	Melanoma	1.36	2.17	2.07
NK1-4	Melanoma	1.25	0.47	0.56
RPM1 5966	Melanoma	1.36	1.48	1.66
A549	Lung carcinoma	4.54**	5.93**	4.76**
A427	Lung carcinoma	1.09	1.31	1.10
9812	Lung carcinoma	1.39	1.22	0.94
HeLa	Cervix carcinoma	55.52***	53.95***	53.58***
EB33	Prostate carcinoma	28.3***	26.11***	26.22***
T24	Bladder carcinoma	1.50	1.76	1.48
PA-1	Ovarian carcinoma	1.61	1.50	1.43
RAJ1	Burkitt lymphoma	1.26	1.06	0.60

Table 2 (con'd.)

Cell Line	Cell Type	Binding ratio[1] of 791T/36 Clone:-		
		Clone 3	Clone 4	Clone 10
(con'd.)				
-	Sheep erythrocytes	1.00	0.56	0.57
73-2295	Canine osteosarcoma	1.10	1.43	1.34
D23	Rat hepatoma	0.78	0.98	0.88
KXD2	Rat hepatoma	1.01	1.12	1.10
Sp4	Rat breast carcinoma	1.25	1.15	1.27

[1] Binding ratio = mean cpm with 791T/36 clone supernatant, divided by mean cpm with P3NS1 spent medium. P3NS1 spent medium gave the same cpm as washing medium. Statistical analysis of the difference between cpm for 791T/36 clone and cpm for P3NS1 medium by the Student t test is indicated by:- *** $P<0.001$, ** $P<0.01$, * $P<0.05$.

[2] 791T, 791 SK, 860 and 870 were from the same patient (M. U.).

[3] 788T and 788 SK were from the same patient (P. R.).

[4] 805T and 805 SK were from the same patient (B. L.).

[5] NT = Not tested.

with osteogenic sarcomas 791T and 788T, HeLa cells and prostate carcinoma EB33, and more weakly reactive with osteogenic sarcomas 805T and 845T, colon carcinomas Ht29 and lung carcinoma A549. No reactivity was observed with 10 different fibroblast lines, three of which were derived from the 791T tumor donor, erythrocytes and mononuclear cells from 10 different individuals, sheep red blood cells, or a variety of cultured human tumor cells (other than those mentioned above). The total number of osteogenic sarcomas positive was four of 10 lines tested, and the proportion of unrelated tumors reacting positively was four out of 22 lines. The anti-791T/36 clones were thus nonreactive to normal host components of the tumor donor, blood group and DR antigens, Forssman antigen or culture artifacts such as adsorbed bovine serum components. On this basis it was concluded that the reactivity was directed toward a tumor-associated antigen which was not shared by all osteogenic sarcomas and not confined to this tumor type. One clone (anti-791T/36 Clone 3) has been selected for further study.

Two 791T-positive clones of anti-791T/48 were subjected to the same extensive testing for reactivity to target cells. Again, the two clones were identical in their reactivity, but this was quite different from that observed with the anti-791T/36 clones (Table 3). Reactivity was again observed with 791T and osteogenic sarcoma 788T cells, but less strong than obtained with anti-791T/36. Conversely, unrelated lines which reacted with anti-791T/36 (HeLa, EB33, A549 and HT29) were negative with anti-791T/48. The anti-791T/48 clones did not react with other control cells (fibroblasts from the tumor donor, erythrocytes and mononuclear cells) so it seemed likely that this hybridoma was detecting another, separate, tumor-associated antigen which was shared by both 791T and 788T. One of the anti-791T/48 clones (anti-791T/48 clone 15) was then selected to evaluate this point further.

Antibodies anti-791T/36 clone 3 and anti-791T/48 clone 15 were purified by affinity chromatography on Protein A linked to Sepharose 4B, and the purified antibodies were labelled with ^{125}I by a chloramine T method (McConahey and Dixon, 1966). The direct binding of the ^{125}I-

Table 3

Cross-Reactivity of Monoclonal Antibodies Against Cell Lines Derived from Different Tumors

Target Cells		Binding Ratio[1] with Monoclonal Antibody[2]			
		Anti-791T/36	Anti-791T/48	SC3982	HRT18/2/3
791T	Osteogenic Sarcoma	26.49***[3]	13.76***	0.61	5.97**
788T	Osteogenic Sarcoma	51.07***	10.08**	0.95	4.43**
888T	Osteogenic Sarcoma	1.08	1.31	1.49	NT
HT29	Colon carcinoma	6.66**	0.99	NT[4]	0.74
HRT18	Colon carcinoma	1.21	0.81	1.21	5.05*
A549	Lung carcinoma	5.39**	1.14	1.25	0.56
A427	Lung carcinoma	1.09	1.64	NT	0.75
EB38	Prostate carcinoma	28.30***	1.40	1.66	1.26
HeLa	Cervical carcinoma	55.52***	1.17	NT	2.54*
SkBr3	Breast carcinoma	1.65	10.94***	NT	NT
74BM	Foetal bone marrow	1.69	2.75*	1.33	2.58*
PA-1	Ovarian carcinoma	1.61	0.90	0.94	0.27
T24	Bladder carcinoma	1.50	0.84	0.90	0.26
HC18	Colon carcinoma	1.61	1.02	NT	3.88*
RPMI 8966	Melanoma	1.16	0.95	0.95	2.58*

[1] Antibody binding detected by uptake of ^{125}I-Protein A on to treated cells. Binding ratio -- mean cpm bound by cells treated with monoclonal antibody -- mean cpm bound by cells treated with P3NS1 spent medium.

[2] Anti-791T/36 and anti-791T/48 were raised against 791T cells. SC 3982 is a coded anti-melanoma monoclonal antibody provided by Dr. S. Ferrone. HRT18/33b was raised against HRT18 cells.

[3] *** $P<0.001$, ** $P<0.01$, * $P<0.05$ (Student t test)

labelled monoclonal antibodies was then tested against 791T, 788T and unrelated cell lines whose reactivity in the indirect ^{125}I Protein A assay was already known (Dawood et al., 1982). The tests with directly labelled antibody were less sensitive than the ^{125}I protein assay since weak cross-reactions were not easy to confirm (e.g., anti-791T/36 against Ht29 and A549), but all of the strongly-reacting lines showed the same qualitative reactivity as in the direct assay. Thus, both anti-791T/36 and anti-791T/48 bound to 791T and 788T cells, and anti-791T/36 bound to HeLa and EB33, but neither antibody bound to cells which were negative by the ^{125}I Protein A test. Also, anti-791T/48 gave weaker reactions with 791T and 788T osteogenic sarcoma cells than did anti-791T/36, so the quantitative difference between the two monoclonal antibodies was to a large extent preserved. Having determined that the respective activities of the two labelled antibodies were essentially unchanged, "cold" antibody inhibition tests were then carried out to determine whether the epitopes they detected were closely *related* or *separate*, as suggested by their different cross-reactivity. It was shown that binding of ^{125}I-labelled anti-791T/36 to 791T, 788T or HeLa cells was inhibited by pretreatment with anti-791T/36 culture supernatant or affinity-purified antibody, but not by equivalent preparations of anti-791T/48. Conversely, labelled anti-791T/48 was inhibited from binding to 791T following incubation of the cells with anti-791T/48 supernatant or purified antibody, but not anti-791T/36. Additional controls were provided by a melanoma monoclonal antibody (coded SC 3892) which did not react with either 791T or 788T, and an anti-rectal carcinoma monoclonal antibody (HRT18/2/336) which reacted with both 788T and 791T. Neither of these control antibodies inhibited the uptake of anti-791T/36 or anti-791/48 by 791T cells. Thus, it was quite clear that the two anti-791T monoclonal antibodies reacted against different epitopes on 791T cells, and also that these epitopes were distinct from a third shared epitope detected by the cross-reactive anti-HRT18/2/336 antibody.

If reactivities can be detected against multiple separate tumor-associated antigens, an important question is to what extent do these murine monoclonal antibodies recognize antigens which are immunogenic in the tumor host? This problem is difficult to resolve, but was partly answered in the case of anti-791T/36 monoclonal antibody. A number of sera from the 791T tumor donor, and also a number of control sera, were screened for reactivity to 791T tumor cells. Some were found to be positive, both for the 791T cells and for control fibroblasts, and others were negative for both tumor and control cells. When tested for the ability to block binding of ^{125}I-labelled anti-791T/36 monoclonal antibody to 791T neither positive nor negative autochthonous host sera showed any consistent inhibitory effect. There was thus no evidence that the anti-791T/36 antibody recognized a 791T-associated antigen also recognized by the tumor host.

It is clear from tests using ^{125}I-labelled antibodies purified by affinity chromatography using Sepharose-Protein A, that the number of antibodies bound per cell is large, suggesting a high frequency of the appropriate epitope. At saturation approximately 1.6×10^6 and 2×10^5 antibodies are bound per 791T target cell using respectively anti-791T/36 and anti-791T/48 monoclonal antibodies. The frequency of common structures such as Concanavalin A-binding sites is around 2×10^7 sites per cell, at least with many experimental tumors, so that the antigenic targets for these two antibodies, particularly the anti-791T/36 monoclonal antibody, represent surface components in sufficient abundance to be amenable to biochemical characterization. At present, it is not known whether the epitopes for these antibodies are expressed individually upon single surface macromolecules or whether they may be represented by repetitive sequences within surface proteins or glycoproteins. Clearly, however, the epitopes for these two anti-osteogenic sarcoma antibodies are expressed upon separate antigenic target structures; not only are their levels of binding at saturation completely different, but in the direct binding assays using radioiodinated antibodies, they did not mutually compete or cross-block in their reaction with their surface antigenic agents (Dawood et al., 1982). There are further differences in the reactivity of these two anti-human osteogenic sarcoma antibodies, such as the fact that anti-791T/36 exhibits complement-dependent cytotoxicity while anti-791T/48 does not.

4. Diagnostic and Therapeutic Uses of Monoclonal Antibodies in Human Tumor Systems

Using osteogenic sarcoma monoclonal antibodies, we will describe several potential uses of these reagents as diagnostic and therapeutic tools.

4.1. Using monoclonal antibodies to define the nature of the cell source

Our group has carried on a series of studies to define the cell source of a variety of related tumors. One such study involved the relationship of a tumor, giant cell tumor of bone which is a relatively benign self-limited tumor, and osteogenic sarcoma, a highly lethal tumor. We discovered that giant cell tumor of bone and osteogenic sarcoma tumors were completely reactive to the limits of the tests, using autologous antisera. The conclusion was that giant cell tumor of bone is really an osteogenic sarcoma but with a vigorous host response (Byers et al., 1975). However, this study underlines one of the many problems which monoclonal antibodies may solve, since it is possible that two separate antigens exist that are chemically very similar but not identical.

4.2. Using monoclonal antibodies to define the nature and extent of metastasis of tumors in vivo

Monoclonal antibodies which define specific tumor antigens can be used in the diagnosis, staging, and therapy of various cancers. For example, monoclonal antibodies could be used to diagnose and stage osteogenic sarcoma. Some 80% or more of the osteogenic sarcoma patients present with solitary primary lesions. The remaining ones have radiologically definable lung metastases at the time of discovery of the disease. Monoclonal antibodies to osteogenic sarcoma could be conjugated to radioisotopic molecules such as ^{125}I or radio-opaque molecules. These ligands can be injected intravenously into patients and the nature of the primary lesion as well as the presence of micromestastasis can be easily ascertained. This information will help to develop a maximally beneficial surgical, immunologic, radiotherapeutic and chemotherapeutic approach to the disease. The detection of micrometastases in the lung may prompt the surgeon to be less aggressive in the removal of the primary. It may, however, warrant the use of earlier and more intensive radiotherapy to the lungs of these patients. Conversely, the absence of micrometastasis may prompt the treating physicians to be aggressive in the removal of the primary and early implementation of adjuvant immunotherapy.

The other tumor type which has been extensively studied using monoclonal antibodies to define the occurrence and cross-reactivity of tumor antigens is malignant melanoma. Studies by Koprowski, et al., are producing a picture similar to that observed with osteogenic sarcoma. Although several monoclonal antibodies have been developed which define antigens common to various lines of human malignant melanomas, these antibodies also react with a few cell lines from other tumor types, and a few cell lines derived from normal tissue.

4.3. Using the monoclonal antibodies therapeutically

Although tumors are able to induce anti-tumor antibodies in their hosts, most data, both in human and animal systems, indicate that these antibodies are relatively ineffective in actually killing the tumors. Work is being directed toward coupling these antibodies to toxic agents, and utilizing the antibodies to bring such agents to the tumors. For example, monoclonal antibodies have been coupled to the chemotherapeutic agent adriamycin (Arnon) by either glutaraldehyde cross-linking between the amino acids of the drug and free amino acid groups or protein, or other similar chemical coupling methods. These complexes have been shown to kill animal tumors, and will provide an important exerimental tool for use in human tumors. It is particularly important with the latter, since there is a large body of literature indicating which chemotherapeutic agent is maximally effective against which tumor type. The chief drawback to all chemotherapy is of course the fact that the toxic effect is not specific, and kills normal cells as well as tumor cells. Such side effects would be vastly reduced if antibody linked chemotherapeutic agents were effective.

A second approach is the use of plant and bacterial toxins to couple to monoclonal anti-tumor antibodies. An example is diphtheria toxin.

This is an acidic globular protein with two chains. The first chain (A chain) interferes with protein synthesis. The second chain (B chain) binds to a specific receptor on the target cell. When the B chain binds, the A chain enters the cell. Once introduced into a target cell, the B chain produces inhibition of protein synthesis and cell death. However, the A chain is only toxic if linked to the B chain. Since the B chain receptor is so wildly distributed on various cells in the body, the toxin normally causes death of the entire organism. However, if the A chain, which is nontoxic extracellularly but only toxic intracellularly, is coupled to an anti-tumor monoclonal antibody, then the resultant combination should be specifically reactive to tumor cells, and lethal only to them. There is a wide range of other toxins which are currently being investigated. To date, the conjugates have been shown to be effective in vitro. After proper animal testing they should be ready for testing in humans.

In summary, therefore, the common theme in these studies is that antigens exist which are found primarily on malignant cells of a certain cell type. Antibodies directed against these antigens, however, react against other malignant and normal cells of different cell types. The important question to resolve is whether the antigens on the other cell types are truly identical in chemical structure to the tumor antigens or represent cross-reacting antigens. A classical example of cross-reacting antigens is the Forssman antigen. The Forssman antigen is an antigen well known in clinical medicine which is found on beef heart and fortuitously reacts with antibodies against *Trepanoma pallidum*, the organism involved in syphilis. However, because the chemical structure of these antigens is closely related but not identical, affinity studies can differentiate between them. Such studies will have to be done with the tumor antigens. The nature of these differences is highly important from a theoretical standpoint, since it provides information about the genetic makeup of normal, as opposed to malignant, cells. From a therapeutic standpoint, however, the requirement for highly specific antibodies with well defined reactivity against tumors has already been met, and monoclonal antibodies, when combined to conventional chemotherapeutic moieties, carry the promise of significant increase in efficacy with significant decrease in side effects. Many laboratories are making ready to use such conjugates in clinical trials in human cancers.

5. References

1. Arnon, R. *Tumor-Associated Antigens and Their Specific Immune Response*, eds. F. Spreafico and R. Arnon, Academic Press, London, 1979, pp. 287-304.

2. Baldwin, R.W., Embleton, M.J., and Price, M.R. Monoclonal antibodies specifying tumour associated antigens and their potential for therapy. In: *Molecular Aspects of Medicine*, Pergamon Press, London, 1981.

3. Bloom, E.T. Further definition by cytotoxicity test of cell surface antigens of Human Sarcoma in culture. *Cancer Res.*, 32, p. 960-967, 1972.

4. Byers, V.S. and Baldwin, R.W. In: *Basic and Clinical Immunology, 3rd Edition.* Eds. H.H. Fudenberg, D.P. Stites, J.L. Caldwell and J.V. Wells, Lange, Los Altos, 1980, pp. 296-312.

5. Byers, V.S. and Johnston, J.O. Antigenic differences among osteogenic sarcoma tumor cells taken from different locations in human tumors. *Cancer Res.*, 37, p. 3173-3183, 1977.

6. Byers, V.S., Levin, A.S., Johnston, J.O., and Hackett, A.J. Quantitative immunofluorescence studies of the tumor antigen bearing cell of Giant Cell Tumor of bone and osteogenic sarcoma. *Cancer Res.*, 35, p. 2520-2531, 1975.

7. Croce, C.M., Linnenbach, A., Hall, W., Steplewski, Z. and Koprowski, H. Production of human hybridomas secreting antibodies to measles virus. *Nature*, 288, p. 488, 1980.

8. Dawood, F., Embleton, M.J., Price, M.R., Byers, V.S. and Baldwin, R.W. *Brit. J. Cancer*, 1982, in press.

9. Embleton, M.J., Gunn, B., Byers, V.S. and Baldwin, R.W. R.W. Antitumour reactions of monoclonal antibody against a human osteogenic-sarcoma cell line. *Brit. J. Cancer*, 43, p. 582, 1981.

10. Hewitt, H.B., Blake, E.R., and Walder, A.S. A critique of the evidence for active host defence against cancer, based on personal studies of 27 murine tumors of spontaneous origin. *Brit. J. Cancer*, 33, p. 241-259, 1976.

11. Köhler, G. and Milstein, C. Continuous cultures of fused cells secreting antibody of predefined specificity. *Nature*, 256, p. 495-497, 1975.

12. McConahey, P.J. and Dixon, F.J. A method of trace iodination of proteins for immunological studies. *Int. Arch. Allergy*, 29, p. 185, 1966.

13. Moore, M. and Hughes, L.A. Circulating antibodies in human connective tissue malignancy. *Brit. J. Cancer*, 28, Suppl. 1, p. 175, 1973.

14. Morton, D.L. and Malmgren, R.A. Human Osteosarcomas: Immunologic evidence suggesting an associated infectious agent. *Science*, 162, p. 1279-1280, 1968.

15. Morton, D.L., Malmgren, R.A., Holmes, E.C. and Ketcham, A.S. Demonstration of antibodies against human malignant melanoma by immunofluorescence. *Surgery*, 64, p. 233-240, 1968.

16. Rosenberg, S., et al. Serologic studies of the antigens on human osteogenic sarcoma. In: *Serologic Analysis of Human Cancer Antigens*, ed. S.A. Rosenberg, Academic Press, London, pp. 93-121, 1980.

17. Woodruff, M.F.A. *The Interaction of Cancer and Host*, Grune and Stratton, New York, 1980.

Chemical Carcinogenesis and Clonal Selection

Wolfgang J. Bühler*) and Norbert Lenz

Fachbereich Mathematik der Johannes Gutenberg-Universitat Mainz

1. Introduction

There are at last two possible ways in which chemical carcinogens can be thought of bringing about the effect of producing cancer tumors. The first is that they are capable of changing cells (in one or several steps) to cells of a different nature: cancer cells. Most mathematical modeling of chemical carcinogenesis centers around this idea. The second possibility is that the changes required to produce cancer cells from normal tissue cells occur spontaneously not under the influence of a chemical substance and that the carcinogen is selectively toxic i.e. kills or severely damages more normal cells than cells that have undergone some or all transformations on the way to becoming cancerous. The latter idea has been exposed in some detail by R. T. Prehn in 1964. While Prehn does not claim that all chemically induced cancers would originate in the way described he pointed out that the proposed clonal selection theory would be consistent with all or most known facts of chemical carcinogenesis and that indeed at least in some cases it might be a mechanism sufficient to explain the facts. In this paper we are trying to model Prehn's theory in an attempt to see how some of the assumptions influence the conclusions and which of the assumptions are crucial.

---

*) Work partly done at the Statistical Laboratory, Univ. of Calif. Berkeley, supported by U. S. Public Health Service grant ESO1299.

2. A first (too) simple model

We assume that normal tissue will have a tendency to preserve a constant number of cells and to recover from insults by e.g. a toxic chemical, eventually restoring the original situation. To simplify mathematics and maybe justified by the large number of cells involved we shall model this aspect deterministically considering a cell density $D(t)$ (which under normal circumstances would be regulated to be close to 1). The change in D brought about by a carcinogen would be proportional to its dose $f(t)$ at time t and the rate of recovery proportional to the "deficiency" $d(t) = 1 - D(t)$. This leads to the differential equation $D'(t) = -\beta_0 f(t) + \rho d(t)$ which with $D(0) = 1$ has solution $d(t) = \beta_0 e^{-\rho t} \int_0^t f(u) e^{\rho u} du$. We further assume that each cell has a small chance of a first mutation generating a clone of transformed cells. Thus the probability for such a clone being started in a short time interval $(t, t+h)$ is assumed to be $\nu_1 D(t) \cdot h + o(h)$. The clone size will then develop according to a birth and death (BAD) process with rates λ_1, μ_1. Denoting by $X_1(t)$ the total number of cells in all the clones of such first order mutants each of these may mutate further generating a second order mutant. The probability for such an event in $(t, t+h)$ be $\nu_2 X_1(t) h + o(h)$ and $X_2(t)$, the number of second order mutants will develop according to a birth and death process with rates λ_2, μ_2. Analogously third, $\cdots$ up to rth mutations and corresponding BAD process populations will be considered. If spontaneous cancers are supposed to be rare we shall have to assume that at least the early stages of transformed cells form subcritical or critical BAD processes i.e. clones that are bound to become extinct. $X_r(t)$ representing cancerous growth would have to behave supercritically though. Let us assume $\lambda_j(t) = \lambda_j$ to be independent of time and $\mu_j(t) = \mu_j + \beta_j f(t)$ with $\lambda_j \leq \mu_j + \nu_{j+1}$ for $j = 1, 2, \cdots, r-1$ and $\lambda_r > \mu_r$ and $\beta_0 \geq \beta_1 \geq \cdots \geq \beta_r$. Looking first at the expected numbers of cells in the various stages we obtain

$$M_1(t) = E X_1(t) = \int_0^t \nu_1 D(u) m_1(u, t) du$$

where

$$m_j(u,t) = \exp\{\int_u^t (\lambda_j - \mu_j(s) - \nu_{j+1})\,ds\}$$

$$= \exp\{(\lambda_j - \mu_j - \nu_{j+1})(t-u) - \beta_j \int_u^t f(s)\,ds\}$$

is the expected size of a birth and death population with rates λ_j, $\mu_j(t) + \nu_{j+1}$ and started at time u. Analogously

$$M_j(t) = E\,X_j(t) = E\,E[X_j(t)\,|\,X_{j-1}(u), 0 \leqslant u \leqslant t]$$

$$= E \int_0^t \nu_j X_{j-1}(u) m_j(u,t)\,du$$

$$= \nu_j \int_0^t M_{j-1}(u) m_j(u,t)\,du$$

for $2 \leqslant j \leqslant r$. Prehn's statement that "variant clones are able to persist for long periods" led us first to assume the processes $X_1, \cdots, X_{r-1}$ to be critical taking into account emigration by mutation, i.e. $\lambda_j = \mu_j + \nu_{j+1}$ for $1 \leqslant j \leqslant r-1$. Without the influence of a carcinogen this would lead to $m_j(u,t) = 1$, $D(t) = 1$ and thus the expected number $M_{r-1}(t)$ of cells in stage $r-1$ (from which tumors can arise by an additional transformation) would be proportional to t^{r-1}. If the carcinogen is applied over a finite time only (i.e. if $f(s) = 0$ for $s > T$ for some T) then again $m_j(u,t) = 1$ for $u > T$ and $j = 1, 2, \cdots, r-1$ and D approaches 1 so fast that we end up with the conclusion that the difference in $M_{r-1}(t)$ between the cases with and without application of carcinogen is of the order t^{r-2} only. The aspect that the number of "additional" tumors that one should expect due to the carcinogenic effect of the chemical is low compared to the number of spontaneous tumors can easily taken care off by assuming the BAD processes to be slightly subcritical rather than critical. A closer look at the assumptions shows however, that the number of "additional" tumors expected is actually negative (since the carcinogen makes $D < 1$ and increases death rates).

3. Attempts to make the model work

One aspect that we have not considered so far is that descendants of a single transformed cell will stay close together with the effect that several clones of cells of type r arising from the same original cell of type 1 will appear and be counted as only one tumor. Thus, given that at time u a cell is transformed into a cell of type 1, all we want to know is the probability that at the later time t it will have descendents forming a detectable tumor. Denoting this probability by $F(u;t)$ we can write down the probability generating function $f(s;t)$ of the number of tumors $Z(t)$ detectable at time t as $f(s;t) = \exp\{-\nu_1 \int_0^t F(u;t)(1-s)\,du\}$, i.e. $Z(t)$ is Poisson distributed with expectation $-\nu_1 \int_0^t F(u;t)\,du$. Here for fixed u the function $F(u,\cdot)$ is a (possibly highly defective) distribution function.

Having identified the distribution of $Z(t)$ as Poisson we can concentrate our attention on the expectation. Now if we consider the situation without the influence of a chemical $F(u,t) = F_0(t-u)$ converging to some value p_0 as $t \to \infty$. Thus $EZ(t) = \nu_1 \int_0^t F_0(t-\tau)\,d\tau \sim \nu_1 p_0 t$. Applying a carcinogen for some finite time only, i.e. assuming $f(s) = 0$ for $s > T$, gives to transformed cells identical conditions as with carcinogen as soon as time is beyond T. Therefore since also $D(s) \to 1$ we have again $EZ(t) = \nu_1 \int_0^t D(u)F(u,t)\,du \sim \nu_1 p_0 t$. A closer look at the difference between the two situations reveals that even

$$\nu_1 \int_0^t [D(u)F(u,t) - F_0(t-u)]\,du$$

$$= \nu_1 \int_0^T [D(u)F(u,t) - F_0(t-u)]\,du$$

$$+ \int_T^t [D(u)-1]F_0(t-u)\,du.$$

Clonal Selection

F_0 being bounded by 1 the latter integral will be bounded by $\int_T^\infty d(u)\, du = \beta_0 \int_T^\infty e^{-\rho u} \int_0^u f(s) e^{\rho s}\, ds = \beta_0 \int_T^\infty e^{-\rho u} \int_0^T f(s) e^{\rho s}\, ds$ which is a finite number.

Thus, in its present setup the model still shares with the setup of the previous section the property that the effect of the carcinogen would be much less than what happens spontaneously anyway. Also what is still not remedied is the fact that the expected number of additional tumors is negative ($D < 1$ means fewer clones are started and increasing death rates in them will leave them with a worse chance to survive into tumors). Actually D is not modeled according to biological reality which says that normal tissue reacts to an insult by e.g. a toxic chemical not just by restoring the old density but by some overreaction which would lead to damped oscillations in $D(t)$. One way to model this is to assume $d(t) = d_0 e^{-\rho(t-u)} \cos(\gamma(t-u))$ if d is started at time u at d_0. Further imagine that f creates at time u the new deficiency $f(u)\, du$ and superimpose to $d(t) = \int_0^t f(u) e^{-\rho(t-u)} \cos(\gamma(t-u))\, du$. Again considering the situation with $f(u)=0$ for $u > T$ we see that for $t > T$ we have $d(t) = \int_0^T f(u) e^{-\rho(t-u)} \cos(\gamma(t-u))\, du$ and thus $|d(t)| \leq e^{-\rho t} \int_0^T e^{\rho u} f(u)\, du$ which goes to zero fast enough to keep the expected number of additional clones that could develop into tumors bounded. Actually the only way within the present framework that may lead out of this difficulty is to introduce a damping factor much slower than $e^{-\rho(t-u)}$; this however seems unrealistic. Consider now applications of a continuous dose $f(u) \equiv c > 0$. This will yield a deficiency $d(t) = c \int_0^t e^{-\rho u} \cos(\gamma u)\, du$ which is positive for all t and converges to $cA = c \int_0^\infty e^{-\rho u} \cos(\gamma u)\, du$. Thus, again, the number of first order clones started will be reduced by application of the chemical. This cannot be counterbalanced by an increase in their probability to develop into a tumor. To be precise: under this model for continuous dose the expected tumor yield would be $EZ(t) \sim \nu_1(1-cA)p_c t$ with p_c being the probability that a first order mutant would eventually produce a tumor if the respective clones were to multiply as BAD processes with rates λ_j and $\kappa_j + c\beta_j$.

There is one further complication which should be built into the model. So far we have taken into account recovery or even an overreaction for normal tissue only. However, if there is increased growth of the tissue one should expect modified clones to participate in it. This can be modelled by assuming $\lambda_j(t) = \lambda_j + \sigma_j d(t)$. Of course, this will not change the fact that an application of a chemical agent for a limited time can only produce a finite expected number of additional first order clones. However, now the probability of developing into a tumor would be increased for all clones not just the additional ones. This effect will be even more clearly expressed when we use a constant $f = A$ (i.e. continuous dose) and assume that $\beta_j - \sigma_j A$ be negative.

4. A different approach

In this section we shall again consider a tissue consisting of cells of types $0, 1, \cdots, r$. We shall assume the numbers $X_0(t), \cdots, X_r(t)$ of cells of these types to develop as BAD processes with intensities $\lambda_j(t)$, $\mu_j(t)$ ($j = 0, 1, \cdots, r$) and with intensity $\nu_j(t)$ of mutation from type j to type $j+1$ ($j = 0, 1, \cdots, r-1$). The vector $M(t)$ of expectations $EX_j(t)$ ($j = 0, 1, \cdots, r$) is then seen to satisfy the differential equation $M'(t) = A(t)M(t)$ where $A(t)$ is the matrix with diagonal $a_j(t) = \lambda_j(t) - \mu_j(t) - \nu_j(t)$ and sub-diagonal $A_{j+1,j}(t) = \nu_j(t)$ and with all other elements equal zero. Here we have set $\nu_r(t) = 0$ for convenience. Given the initial condition $M(0) = m$ this differential equation can be solved explicitly if the eigenvalues of $A(t)$ are all different and the system of eigenvectors of $A(t)$ does not depend on t. If we define matrices $C, \tilde{C}$, by

$$C_{ij} = 0 \quad \text{for } i < j$$

$$= 1 \quad \text{for } i = j$$

$$= \frac{\nu_j \cdots \nu_{i-1}}{(a_{j+1}-a_j)\cdots(a_i-a_j)} \quad \text{for } i > j$$

$$\tilde{C}_{ij} = 0 \quad \text{for } i < j$$

$$= 1 \quad \text{for } i = j$$

$$= \frac{\nu_j \cdots \nu_{i-1}}{(a_j-a_i)\cdots(a_{i-1}-a_i)} \quad \text{for } i > j$$

and let D be the diagonal matrix whose elements are the eigenvalues a_j of A then the relations $AC = CD$, $\tilde{C}A = D\tilde{C}$, $C^{-1}A = DC^{-1}$ are easily verified. It follows that the rows of $\tilde{C}$ are proportional to those of C^{-1}. By virtue of the 1's in the diagonals of both matrices this implies $\tilde{C} = C^{-1}$ and thus $A(t) = C(t)D(t)C^{-1}(t)$. If C is independent of t (which is the case if and only if $\nu_j(t)[\lambda_{j+1}(t)-\lambda_j(t)-\mu_{j+1}(t)+\mu_j(t)-\nu_{j+1}(t)-\nu_j(t)]^{-1}$ does not depend on t) then we obtain the solution $M(t) = CH(t)C^{-1}m$ where $H(t)$ is diagonal with entries $\exp\{\int_0^t a_j(s)\,ds\}$. This can be written as $M_j(t) =$

$$\sum_{l=0}^{j} m_l \nu_l \nu_{l+1} \cdots \nu_{j-1}$$

$$\cdot \sum_{i=l}^{j} \left\{ (a_l-a_i)\cdots(a_{i-1}-a_i)(a_{i+1}-a_i)\cdots(a_j-a_i)\exp\left[-\int_0^t a_i(s)\,ds\right] \right\}^{-1}.$$

To illustrate the use of this formula without too extensive notation assume $r = 2$ and $\nu_j, \mu_j = \lambda_j = \lambda$ for $j = 0, 1, \lambda_2 = \Lambda > M = \mu_2$ all independent of time. Further put $f \equiv 0$. Then $M(t)$ can be written as

$$M_0 = a_{00}(t) m_0$$

$$M_1(t) = a_{10}(t) m_0 + a_{11}(t) m_1$$

$$M_2(t) = a_{20}(t) m_0 + a_{21}(t) m_1 + a_{22}(t) m_2$$

with $a_{00}(t) = e^{-\nu_0 t}$, $a_{10}(t) = \nu_0(e^{-\nu_0 t} - e^{-\nu_1 t})/(\nu_1 - \nu_0)$, $a_{11}(t) = e^{-\nu_1 t}$

$$a_{20}(t) = \nu_0 \nu_1 \Big\{ e^{-\nu_0 t}/[(\nu_0 - \nu_1)(\Lambda - M + \nu_0)]$$

$$+ e^{-\nu_1 t}/[(\nu_1 - \nu_0)(\Lambda - M + \nu_1)] + e^{(\Lambda - M)t}/[(\Lambda - M + \nu_0)(\Lambda - M + \nu_1)] \Big\}$$

$a_{21}(t) = \nu_1(e^{(\Lambda - M)t} - e^{-\nu_1 t})/(\Lambda - M + \nu_1)$, $a_{22}(t) = e^{(\Lambda - M)t}$. If we assume that the dose pattern f of the chemical induced increases death intensities by $\beta_j f(t)$, $\beta_0 > \beta_1 > \beta_2 > 0$ we see that time independence of C requires f to be constant. With a piecewise constant f the solution can be obtained in steps. We assume further that recovery of the tissue will be achieved by an equal increase in λ_j by $\lambda(t)$ for all j which will not disturb the time independence of C. Let there be a time T after which f vanishes. Let $D = \exp\left\{ \int_0^T f(s) \, ds \right\}$ and $G = \exp\left\{ \int_0^t \lambda(s) \, ds \right\}$. Then we can again solve the differential equation and approximate its solution for t large as compared to T by $\hat{M}_0(t) = a_{00}(t) \hat{m}_0$, $\hat{M}_1(t) = a_{10}(t) \hat{m}_0 + a_{11}(t) \hat{m}_1$, $\hat{M}_2(t) = a_{20}(t) \hat{m}_0 + a_{21}(t) \hat{m}_1 + a_{22}(t) \hat{m}_2$ where $\hat{m}_j = m_j G D^{-\beta_j}$. G can now be determined in such a way as to make $\hat{M}_0(t) + \hat{M}_1(t) + \hat{M}_2(t) = M_1(t) + M_2(t) + M_3(t)$. This allows us to look at $\hat{M}_2(t)/M_2(t) = G(a_{20} D^{-\beta_0} m_0 + a_{21} D^{-\beta_1} m_1 + a_{22} D^{-\beta_2} m_2)(a_{20} m_0 + a_{21} m_1 + a_{22} m_2)^{-1}$ which can be thought of as a measure for the carcinogenic efficiency of the chemical given a total dose of log D. We see that $\hat{M}_2(t)/M_2(t)$ is 1 if $\beta_0 = \beta_1 = \beta_2$ i.e. if toxicity is not selective and that it approaches $[(M_0(t) + M_1(t) + M_2(t))/M_2(t)][a_{20}/(a_{00} + a_{10} + a_{20})]$ as D or β_0 become large. With $\Lambda > M$ and small mutation rates $a_{20}/(a_{00}+a_{10}+a_{20})$ is close to unity. Thus a high dose of a severely (and selectively) toxic chemical would turn almost the whole tissue cancerous. This limiting case obviously is beyond biological reality.

5. Remarks

The decisive differences between the model discussed in section 3 and the previous discussion are the facts that firstly the number of normal cells (type 0) is not any more treated deterministically (and in fact as practically infinite) entailing an unlimited stream of first order mutants and secondly that intermediate clones now are treated as critical without taking into account mutation such that mutation actually will turn them subcritical ($\lambda_j < \mu_j+\nu_j$). It is probably the second of these facts that is essential and of course we could have handled the previous situation in a corresponding way. Whereas so far we have not tried to check the model against biological reality represented by data on tumor occurances it is our feeling that at least qualitatively the mathematical conclusions may be seen as supporting or at least not contradicting Prehn's ideas. We are aware that computations with data such as those coming from experiments with dose fractionation or with a succession of different chemicals would be likely to point out deficiencies of the model and force us to appropriately modify it.

6. References

[1] Harris, T. E.: *The theory of branching processes* (Springer-Verlag; Berlin, 1963)

[2] Prehn, R. T.: A clonal selection theory of chemical carcinogenesis. *J. Nat. Cancer Inst.* 32, 1-17 (1964).

[3] Puri, P. S.: On the homogeneous birth-and-death process and its integral. *Biometrika* 53, 61-71 (1966).

Avenue to Understanding the Mechanism of Radiation Effects: Extended Serial Sacrifice Experimental Methodology

Jerzy Neyman

Statistical Laboratory
University of California, Berkeley, CA 94720

1. Introduction

The present paper was intended for delivery at the Workshop at the Institute for Energy Analysis, Oak Ridge Associated Universities, held in October 1979. I regret that I was not able to attend this Workshop. However, I did attend the earlier Workshop at the same Institute held in September 1977, the *Proceedings* of which have been just published [1]. I find these *Proceedings* very interesting, especially because of what I learned from experimenting biologists. This confirms my conviction that health effects of radiation is a highly interdisciplinary domain. Progress in this domain depends upon close collaboration between interested biologists-experimentors, on the one hand, and of equally interested statisticians, on the other. Here is an illustration.

There were 19 papers presented at the Workshop of 1977. Nine of them have titles including the words "competing risks". A substantial part of the statistical community is familiar with this term, particularly in connection with the "risk" of dying from this or that specified "cause". E.g. in certain conditions thymic lymphoma is a "strong competitor" of reticulum cell sarcoma, etc.

Here, then, the term "competing risk" refers to phenomena supposed to develop in the bodies of living organism, the phenomena that are the subject of experimental and theoretical studies. However, when reading the contributions of R. J. Michael Fry, Everett Staffeldt and Sylvanus A.

Tyler, [1, pp. 361-366], and of J. M. Holland, [1, pp. 367-370], I learned of a very different competition of risks. This competition is going on not in the bodies of experimental animals, but in the laboratories in which the dead animals are necropsied!

It appears that some diseases are easily detected by "gross examination", but some others are not and require the use of microscopes. Obviously, this kind of competition and its results are not helpful in the efforts to understand the mechanism of radiation effects on health and I am appreciative of the following insistence of Holland:

> It is important to compare cohorts . . . with respect to specific disease states . . . it is essential that each animal receive the same qualitative and quantitative necropsy . . . fixed within examination protocol. Essential features of this protocol include a listing of all major organs and tissues . . .

Hopefully, Dr. Holland's insistence in 1977 became a general rule in 1979. His "protocol" is mentioned in Chapter IV of this paper.

In my contribution to the Workshop of 1977, I expressed the view that the concept of the "cause of death" is not useful and should be abandoned. In consequence the many theories of competing risks became uninteresting. Realistic studies of health effects of exposure to any kind of possibly noxious agent depend upon the availability of data on "all major organs and tissues" as insisted by Holland.

The focus of the present paper is intended to be on happenings in the organisms of irradiated experimental animals. The thinking on this subject, my own and of other authors, evolved substantially during the years that elapsed. Some phases of this evolution are described below, including certain interesting experimental findings. My hope is that this description will create an appropriate perspective on the importance of the serial sacrifice methodology invented by Arthur C. Upton in 1969 [2].

2. Evolution in Studies of Health-related Effects of Radiation

1. *My first contact with the problem.* My first contact with the problem of effects of irradiation on health goes back to the fall of 1958. In my capacity as a visitor at the National Institute of Health (NIH) I was asked to examine the literature relating to the existence of a threshold below which the irradiation could have no adverse health effects. At the time it was already commonly believed that adverse health effects of irradiation include cancer. The initiation of cancer was attributed to vaguely understood "mutations" supposed to occur in cells of living tissues.

Of the literature I read at the NIH the most relevant appeared in two interconnected papers, both published in *Science*, Vol. 128 (1958). The first of the two papers, authored by M. P. Finkel (pp. 637-641) describes experiments intended to estimate the irradiation threshold. The second paper, by A. M. Brues (pp. 693-699) describes theoretical reasons for the author's conviction that a threshold of irradiation carcinogenesis must exist. Briefly, Dr. Brues' reasons were that the mechanism of carcinogenesis must involve not just one but at least two stages, each involving mutation. Of these several stages, only the last is ascribed to irradiation. The earlier, the "precancerous stages" had to be ascribed to some other agents.

The reader will notice that the above description implies a ramification of the problem of carcinogenesis, irradiation -- yes, but in addition there had to be some other noxious agents, presumably chemical. In these circumstances it was natural for me to search for literature on experimental evidence of chemical carcinogenesis. This I found in several publications describing impressive experiments performed by M. B. Shimkin and M. Polissar, published in 1954, 1955 and 1958 in the *Journal of the National Cancer Institute*. The experiments were concerned with one particular chemical, urethane.

The study of the Shimkin and Polissar experiments may be labeled as the second phase of my acquaintance with carcinogenesis. The third phase was especially concerned with one question posed by Dr. Brues, namely, whether the mechanism of carcinogenesis is one-staged or multi-staged. Influenced by the work of Shimkin and Polissar, the concern was with the urethane carcinogenesis (or "tumorogenesis") and, specifically, with the question of an experimental design that could provide an unambiguous resolution of the dilemma: one-stage or multi-stage?

The results of this study, comprising three interconnected papers, are published in the *Proc. Fifth Berkeley Symposium Math. Stat. and Prob.* Vol. 4 (1967) [Univ. of California Press, Berkeley, CA 94720]. The three papers in question were authored by Shimkin *et al* (pp. 707-720), by White *et al* (pp. 721-744) and by Neyman and Scott (pp. 745-776). The studies included a large number of experiments, conducted and analyzed in terms of contemporary biological "state-of-the-art", appeared consistent with the multi-stage hypothesis of carcinogenesis. It seemed appropriate to act on the assumption that the true mechanism of urethane tumorogenesis is a multi-stage mutation mechanism.

When I was writing the above conclusion, the old Latin saying came to mind: "Oh fallacem hominem spem!" The disenchantment occurred a few years later when Margaret R. White completed her experiment intended to verify a particular assumption (or "presumption") of the earlier "state-of-the-art". Briefly and roughly, Margaret White used an innovative method to test two "classical" presumptions. One of them was that urethane injected into mice is eliminated from their bodies in a very short time, that, for practical purposes, could be considered instantaneous. The second classical presumption tested by Miss White was that the speed of eliminating urethane from the bodies of mice does not depend upon the dose injected. The innovative method of Miss White consisted in using "labeled" urethane.

The molecule of urethane includes three atoms of carbon. In her experiment Miss White used two kinds of labeled urethane, termed "C-labeled" and "E-labeled". In each case one particular atom of carbon was replaced by a radionucleide ^{14}C.

Miss White's results are published in two related papers, both in the

Proc. of the Sixth Berkeley Symposium, Vol. 4 (1972) [Univ. of California Press, Berkeley, CA 94720]. The biological aspect of the study is described by Miss White (pp. 287-308). The part oriented towards statistical readers is in the paper of C. Guillier (pp. 309-316). The general conclusion of the two papers is that the speed of elimination of urethane from the bodies of mice depends strongly on the dose injected and, in consequence, that the mechanism of urethane tumorogenesis is likely to be a one-stage mechanism.

Some details of the above evolutionary phases will be found in the next chapter. As of now, it is appropriate to point out that the process of evolution was due to excessive reliance of particular research workers on preconceptions which changed from one phase to the next, when they were found unjustified. Compared to these, the serial sacrifice experimental methodology appears to depend on the least amount of preconceived ideas. Its aim is to find what are the facts. However, it does need certain extensions.

3. Some Details of Particular Evolutionary Phases.

(i) *A. M. Brues.* The following passage is reproduced from the article of Dr. A. M. Brues quoted earlier:

> There are many examples of induction of malignant disease through mechanisms which are clearly indirect -- that is, where irradiation of a cell can be shown not to be a critical factor . . . There is a large body of evidence indicating that the malignant transformation occurs after a sequence of 'precancerous' stages has taken place. The most widely observed example is in the development of skin cancer, which, in whatever way it is produced, is likely to be preceded by various types of benign atrophic or hyperplastic states; in experimental studies it most often develops in a benign papilloma.

(ii) *M. B. Shimkin and M. J. Polissar.* While the above quote illustrates indirect documentation of Dr. Brues, the following somewhat longish quote describes the Shimkin and Polissar efforts to obtain experimental evidence of the happenings in the lungs of mice following the injection of a single dose of urethane. The quote reproduces a passage in reference [3].

8.1. *Shimkin and Polissar data.* Table I and figure 2 represent the experimental results of Shimkin and Polissar. For purposes of the present section, only the last column of the table is needed. This gives the estimated average number $\zeta(T)$ of tumor nodules in the lungs of mice all given the same dose of urethane 1 mg/gm BW, and sacrificed at varying times after the injection specified in the first column ... Figure 2 shows a plot of $\zeta(T)$ against T. It is seen that, while the unavoidable random fluctuation of $\zeta(T)$ are quite noticeable, the convergence of $\zeta(T)$ to an asymptotic value is pronounced. Inspection of figure 2 suggests strongly that, if more than one series of mice were available, each series with a different dose D of urethane administered in a single injection, then counts of tumors made after some 20 weeks might reasonably be considered as empirical counterparts of $\zeta(+\infty)$, and used for the verification of the one stage mutation hypothesis.

The experimental data resulted from microscopic examination of slices of the lungs of mice -- a methodology that many other experimentalists did not use.

(iii) *One-stage or multistage?* The Shimkin and Polissar findings illustrated above refer to temporal changes in two characteristics of the lungs of mice: the abundance of presumed "first mutant" cells, including the "hyperplastic foci" and of tumors. The presumed first mutant cells and the foci increase up to about 49 days and then decline to zero. Thus, these cells and their foci must be "benign". The tumors begin to be noticeable on the 28th day after the urethane injection. Then their abundance increases rapidly and, after about 50 days, becomes stabilized. The question is whether the noted changes in the "benign" cells and of tumors are two unrelated consequences of the injected urethane, or do the "benign" cells represent the "precancerous" growth as anticipated by Brues? Another

TABLE I

Counts of Cells, of Hyperplastic Foci, and of Tumors in Lungs of Mice After Shimkin and Polissar [12].

Days after Urethane	Estimated Mean Number of:			
	Cells per Square (106.3 sq. micra)	Presumed First Mutants per Square	Foci per Lung	Tumors per Lung
0	0.73	0.00	—	—
1	0.85	0.12	—	—
3	0.92	0.19	—	—
7	1.11	0.38	—	—
14	1.02	0.29	294	—
21	1.35	0.62	450	—
28	1.57	0.84	390	15.5
38	—	—	610	—
49	1.33	0.60	450	37.3
84	1.20	0.47	260	34.8
105	—	—	200	35.2
133	—	—	83	35.7

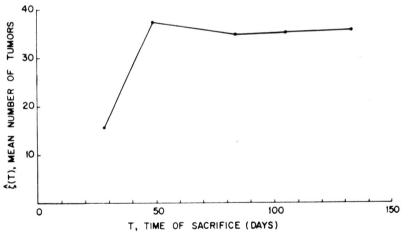

FIGURE 2

Estimated mean number of tumor nodules per lung.
Each mouse received same dose of urethane 1 mg/gm BW,
sacrificed at varying times T after injection.
Data from Shimkin and Polissar [7].

important question is: how to design an experiment that could answer the question unambiguously?

Regretfully, in their work just described, Shimkin and Polissar made their counts of the two kinds of objects independently from each other. Also the amount of time and labor was too high to repeat the experiment. The practical possibilities appeared limited to experiments with varying doses of urethane and with counts of tumors performed with the naked eye as they appear on the surface of the lungs of the sacrificed mice. The basic idea of the many experiments actually performed was that, if the mechanism of carcinogenesis is one-stage, then the ultimate crop of tumors must be independent of the time pattern at which a given dose of urethane is injected, whether in a single injection or in several equal fractions administered a few days apart. On the other hand, if the true mechanism is multistage and if the interval between the successive injections happens to be close to the time of the maximum of "precancerous" cells, then the fractionated administration of a given dose would be expected to result in an increased number of tumors.

Briefly, the many experiments performed varied in many respects, including the strains of mice, some of which proved very variable in their response. However, one question appeared to have been answered unambiguously: The crop of tumors counted was found to depend sharply on the time pattern of administering the same total dose of urethane. Specifically, when a fixed total dose D of urethane, measured in milligrams per gram of body weight of the mice, was administered either at once or in equal fractions over about a month, the fractionated administration resulted in a very substantial *decrease* in the total number of tumors counted.

In accordance with the contemporary ideas about the effectiveness of urethane, the conclusion reached was that the mechanism of the urethane tumorogenesis cannot be a one-stage mechanism. The credit for questioning this conclusion and for performing an experiment to test one of its basic assumptions belongs to Margaret R. White.

(iv) *Is the number of initial urethane tumorogenic events proportional to the dose injected?* The two pages of graphs reproduced from the article of Guillier already quoted seem to be the most informative way to summarize the findings of Miss White.

The page on the left, Guillier's figures 2 and 3, illustrate Miss White's results obtained using the C-labelled urethane. The other page, with figures 4 and 5, refers to E-labelled urethane. The curves in all the figures, marked by different symbols, refer to five replicates of a specified experiment. In each case, the ordinate of a point on the curve represents the percentage of the total number of injected ^{14}C atoms that, after so many hours since the injection, still remain not removed from the bodies of the mice. At time zero, this percentage is 100%. Subsequently, as hours go by, the proportion of unremoved ^{14}C atoms decreases, first slowly, then faster, but eventually approaching a horizontal asymptote. The height of this asymptote reflects the proportion of the injected atoms ^{14}C that failed to be eliminated through the process studied, namely through exhaling. The remaining ^{14}C atoms may have been eliminated otherwise, perhaps in urine, or may have been incorporated in the bodies of mice, perhaps in their bones, etc.

The essential details of the four graphs are: (a) the ^{14}C atoms of the E-labelled urethane are exhaled more slowly than those of the C-labelled urethane, which documents the fact that molecules of the urethane must have been metabolized, and (b) that the speed of the elimination of urethane is sharply dependent on the size of the dose injected. Figures 2 and 4 correspond to the dose of 1 mg/g of the body weight of the mice while Figures 3 and 5 correspond to the dose of one eighth of one milligram.

Note: Miss White's experiment included a substantial number of different dosages of urethane. The lowest was 0.125 mg/g. Next there were dosages 0.25 mg/g, 0.50 mg/g, 1.00 mg/g, 1.20 mg/g and 1.40 mg/g. With the two heaviest dosages some mice failed to survive the experiment. The results obtained with one-half and with one-quarter of a milligram were intermediate to those reproduced by Guillier, indicating the same

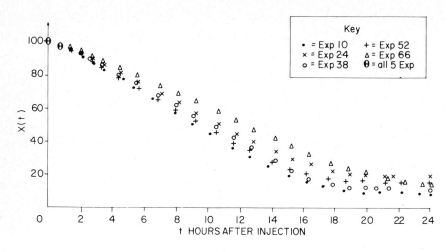

Figure 2

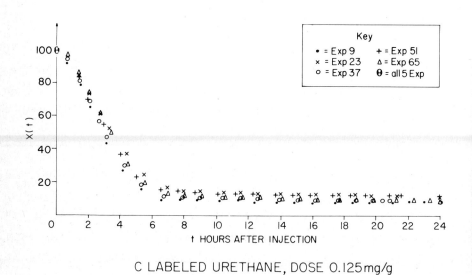

Figure 3

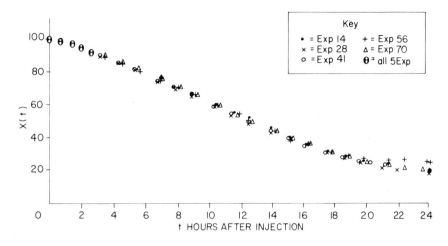

Figure 4

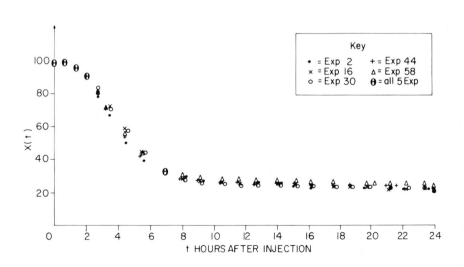

Figure 5

general patterns.

The conclusion implied by Miss White's results is unambiguous; with large doses of the injected urethane the entities within the bodies of mice that govern the exhaling (enzymes?) must have become temporarily overwhelmed. In other words, the molecules of the urethane (or their metabolites) spend more time in the bodies of mice if injected in larger doses and can produce relatively more "initial" tumorogenic effects than they could with small doses. This is confirmed by other details of Miss White's experiment.

What are the implications? What about the realism of the conclusion of the earlier phase that the urethane tumorogenesis cannot be one-stage?

Margaret White's findings contradict this conclusion.

4. Serial Sacrifice Methodology: A Direct Approach to Health Effects of Irradiation

(i) *Analogy with insurance problems.* The empirical study of effects of irradiation presupposes two groups of animals (say mice). One group is subjected to irradiation (say "experimentals") and the other is not (say "controls"). We have here an analogy with insurance related studies conducted for particular groups of the population, each group characterized by some specific conditions of life and employment. Such groups may be exemplified by school teachers, office workers and coal miners.

A question of interest may be whether a single set of actuarial tables would be appropriate to use for all the three population groups mentioned. This would be the case if age dependent death and sickness rates for teachers, office workers and coal miners were approximately the same. Here, it is easy to guess that the rates for miners are likely to be different. But are they? And what about school teachers and office workers?

In order to answer these and many similar questions it is unavoidable to perform studies of "cohorts". Such studies are actually performed using the health and mortality records accumulated in various institutions such as clinics serving various occupational groups, etc. In order to be really reliable, the health records must confirm with Dr. Holland's "protocol" (See Introduction) complete with all of its trimmings. A brief description of findings is as follows.

(ii) *Stability periods.* While particular occupational population groups exist with very different rates of death and sickness, the age related changes in these rates calculated for adults are relatively slow. For example, the year to year changes in death rates, etc. are so small that some tables used in practice gave rates for periods of 5 years. In the following, periods of this kind, with negligible changes in the rates of interest, will be called "stability periods". The determination of the length of stability periods is made using empirical data and taking into account the purpose of the tables.

The reader will realize that such determination, as well as the definition of "adult ages" must be somewhat subjective.

(iii) *Typical questions.* For purposes of the present chapter it is very important to be clear about the typical questions that need to be answered in insurance related studies for specified occupational groups constructed for the adopted stability periods. Here are three questions.

Question 1 How frequently do coal miners die between the ages 40 and 45 while suffering from two specified diseases, say leukemia and influenza?

Question 2 How frequently are coal miners 40 years of age suffering from two diseases combined, namely from leukemia and influenza?

Question 3 refers to coal miners of the category specified in question 2. *Question 3* reads: how frequently do such coal miners die before reaching age 45? More generally, how frequently the coal miners of the same category change their health characteristics before they are 45, perhaps recovering from influenza or developing pneumonia, etc.?

Given good health services organized by the coal miners union, all these three questions can be answered without much trouble. The computable rates are used both for purposes of insurance and, not infrequently, for progress in medical diagnosis. Finally these rates are a "must" in the process of comparing danger in various fields of employment. The reader will realize that just such rates are an emphatic *must* in an experimental study of irradiation effects on mice. The question is whether, and if so, what experimental design could provide Dr. Holland's protocol data for computing rates answering questions similar to the above questions 1, 2, and 3, this both for the experimental and for the control mice.

(iv) *How to answer the three questions for mice?* After establishing the stability periods for mice (and this may require some special experimentation), and granting a satisfactory observance of Holland's "protocol", questions of type 1 are easily answered.

One begins by sorting the mice, separately the experimentals and the controls, that are alive at the beginning of each stability period and count them separately for each period. During any given period some of the mice alive at the beginning will die. Thus, autopsies performed using Dr. Holland's protocol will indicate those having particular combinations of pathological characteristics. This will provide the data for computing the rates. With a detailed protocol, most of the rates will be zero.

Now, let us see whether strict adherance to Dr. Holland's protocol is sufficient to answer questions of type 2. In order to answer this question, one has to know the number of mice *alive* at the beginning of a given stability period and, at that time, having a specified combination of pathological states. However, the establishment of any such combination of pathological states requires detailed autopsies. Obviously, in order to be able to answer the question of type 2, the only way is to take a sample of mice alive at the indicated moment, to "sacrifice" them and to perform the autopsies. This has to be done for each adopted stability period. The necessity of such "serial sacrifices" has been first realized by *Dr. Arthur C. Upton in 1969 [2].* It was Upton who organized a serial sacrifice experiment at the Oak Ridge National Laboratory. To begin with, the chief experimentor was Upton himself. Later, when Upton left the Laboratory, the experiment was completed by Dr. John B. Storer.

(v) *Question 3: an extension of the Upton methodology is needed.*

Question 3 refers to mice alive at the beginning of any stability period and having at that time a known set of pathological characteristics. The question asks for a documented prognosis of the changes in the health characteristics to be expected during the stability period in question.

The reader will realize that the serial sacrifice methodology does not provide data sufficient to formulate the prognosis. Consider a category of mice alive at the beginning of a stability period and having at that time some marks of "precancerous growth" of the kind discussed by Dr. Brues (See Chapter III). One of the possible changes in the state of health of such mice may be the initiation of a malignant growth, but not necessarily. The actual happenings can be observed by sacrificing a sample of the mice in question at the end of the stability period and by performing autopsies in accordance with the Holland protocol. However, in order to be able to compute the rate of interest, it is necessary to have a methodology for determining the frequency with which the mice alive at the beginning of the stability period are marked by the presence of "precancerous growth" without killing these mice.

The conclusion is that the Upton methodology needs an extension. A diagnostic procedure is needed with an efficiency at least approximating the protocol of Dr. Holland, but not requiring the killing or even hurting of these mice. Could something like Bruce Ames' discovery be helpful?

Acknowledgements

This paper was prepared using the facilities of the Statistical Laboratory with partial support from the Office of Naval Research (ONR N00014 75 C 0159), and the National Institute of Environmental Health Sciences (2 R01 ES01299-16). The opinions expressed are those of he author.

References

1. "Environmental Biological Hazards and Competing Risks," Proceedings of a Workshop held at the Institute for Energy Analysis, Oak Ridge Associated Universities, Oak Ridge, TN 37830, U. S. A., 7-8 September 1977, *Environmental International*, Volume 1, Number 6 (1978).

2. Upton, A. C., *et al.*, "Quantitative Experimental Study of Low-Level Radiation Carcinogenesis," *Radiation-Induced Cancer*, International Atomic Energy Agency, Vienna, 1969, pp. 425-438.

3. Neyman, J. and Scott, E. L., "Statistical aspect of the problem of carcinogenesis," *Proceedings of the Fifth Berkeley Symposium on Mathematical Statistics and Probability*, Volume IV (1967), pp. 745-776. University of California Press, Berkeley, CA 94720.

Short-term Tests Used to Detect Mutagens and their Effects in Body Fluids

Renae Magaw and Joyce McCann

Biology and Medicine Division
Lawrence Berkeley Laboratory
Berkeley, CA 94720

1. Introduction

It is likely that most human cancers are caused by both natural and man-made chemical mutagens and by radiation (for discussion of the somatic mutation theory of cancer, see reference 1). Mutagens may also play a role in causing heritable effects in humans (e.g. some birth defects and the gradual accumulation in the human gene pool of subtle, but essentially irreversible deleterious mutations). In the last 10 years, increasing awareness of the importance of environmental factors has led to greater emphasis on prevention of these effects and to attempts to minimize human exposure to hazardous chemicals (for general discussion see reference 2).

A number of "short-term" testing methods for detecting potential chemical carcinogens and mutagens have emerged from the diverse areas of cancer biochemistry, nucleic acid research, genetics, and molecular and cell biology. Over 100 assays have been identified which use a variety of cell types *in vitro*, from bacteria and phage to human cells, as well as tests that can be done directly in animals or people (3).

We will discuss here the short-term tests which can be used to detect mutagens or genetic damage in whole animals by examination of body fluids and bone marrow. This application of short-term tests is of particular interest since body fluids from humans (for additional review see reference

4), such as patients undergoing drug therapy or workers exposed to chemicals in industry, can be analyzed. The presence of mutagens or genetic damage in body fluids are also endpoints, possibly related to cancer- induction, that can be measured directly in animals undergoing the carcinogenesis process and used to resolve issues of comparability between short-term tests and animal cancer tests.

2. Overview of Short-term Tests that Use Body Fluids

Body fluids that have been examined include feces (5, 6, 7, 8), bile (9, 10), milk or breast fluids (11, 12), gastric juice (13, 14, 15), blood (16, 17), semen (18, 19) and urine (20, 21, 22, 23). The presence of chemical mutagens in these body fluids can be detected using a variety of mutagenesis test methods. One can also detect cytogenetic effects of mutagens in peripheral blood lymphocytes, and in developing erythrocytes in bone marrow. Morphological sperm abnormalities can be examined in semen. The major assays that have been used are described below.

A. Direct Detection of Mutagens

The basic technique used in these assays involves treatment of an animal (or human) with a test chemical, removal of the body fluid of interest, and assay for the presence of mutagens. The test organisms used to detect mutagenic activity cover a wide range from bacteria, to mammalian cells, to other eukaryotic organisms such as yeast. Bacteria and yeast are the most commonly used. We describe below three test systems using these indicator organisms.

i). The *Salmonella*Test (24)

This is the most widely used method for direct detection of mutagens in body fluids. Several different strains of *Salmonella* bacteria are used. They have been altered from the wild type by genetic manipulation so that they are particularly sensitive to being mutated by a wide variety of different types of mutagens. These 'tester strains also contain one of several different mutations which make the bacteria unable to synthesize the essential amino acid, histidine. Therefore, they cannot grow unless histidine is added to the growth medium. One does a *Salmonella* test (or 'Ames test') by first growing up a culture of bacteria in the presence of histidine; then plating out in a Petri dish about a hundred million bacteria with the test chemical and a small amount of histidine. (For some chemical mutagens, cell growth is required for mutagenesis).

Figure 1 illustrates the type of result seen when the chemical mutagen is placed on a paper disk, and allowed to diffuse out into the agar. The chemical will, at random, interact with the chromosome in each bacterium, and at a concentration where the chemical is not overly toxic, it can cause a mutation in the histidine gene that will revert it back to the normal form. In each bacterium where this occurs, the cell will begin to grow and divide. After a 2 day incubation period, a visible 'revertant colony' will form. The number of colonies formed indicates the mutagenic potential of the test chemical. An homogenate of mammalian tissue (usually rat liver) is usually also added to the Petri dish to incorporate an aspect of mammalian metabolism into the assay. This is an essential part of the assay because most chemicals that cause mutations are not active as they exist in the environment, and must be metabolically transformed into active chemical species.

In the case of body fluid assays the test chemical and the liver homogenate are replaced by a sample of the body fluid. Mutagens in the body fluid as it is obtained from an animal are often at concentrations below the detectable limit of the mutagenesis assay. Therefore, the sample is usually concentrated before analysis. Figure 2 illustrates a typical dose-response curve from a "plate incorporation" assay (slightly different from the "spot-test" shown in Figure 1) in which the mutagenic activity of urine from cigarette smokers is indicated.

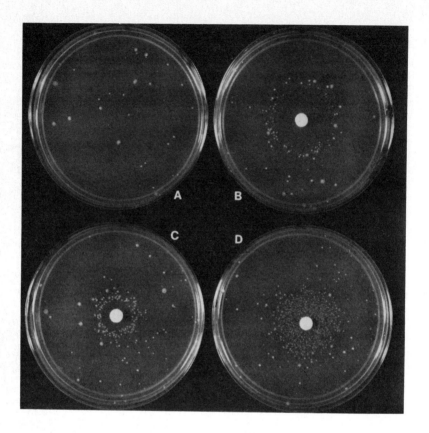

Figure 1. The *Salmonella* spot test. Each petri plate contains, in a thin overlay of top agar, the tester strain TA98, and in the case of plates C and D, a rat liver microsomal activation system. Mutagens were applied to 6 mm filter paper discs which were then placed in the center of each plate: (A) spontaneous revertants, (B) furylfuramide (AF-2) (1 μg), (C) aflatoxin B_1 (1 μg), and (D) 2-aminofluorene (10 μg). Mutagen induced revertants appear as a ring of colonies around each disc. (Adapted from Figure 2 in Ames et al (24)).

ii). The Fluctuation Test (25, 26)

The fluctuation test can be used with many test organisms, including yeast and fungi, as well as bacteria. Very weak mutagens can be detected by this procedure. The principal of mutant detection in this assay is similar to that described above for the *Salmonella* assay. Cells that require an

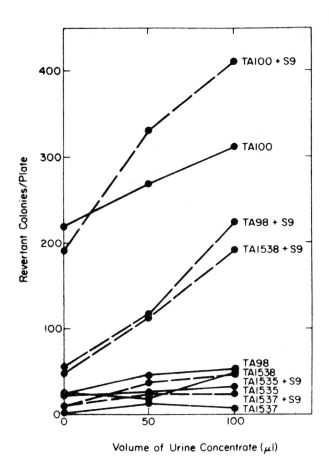

Figure 2. Mutagenicity of compounds in a smokers urine. Urine samples were collected during one day, concentrated, and tested in the *Salmonella* plate incorporation assay with and without metabolic activation (S9). Mutagenic activity is indicated when the urine concentrate is plated with tester strains TA100, TA98 and TA1538. There is no activity with the other tester strains, TA1535 and TA1537. (Adapted from Figure 1 in Yamasaki and Ames (20)).

essential nutrient for growth are treated with the test chemical, or body fluid, and diluted to very low concentrations. They are then distributed among a large number of tubes (usually 100) containing medium with a limiting amount of the required nutrient. After incubation for 3-4 days the number of tubes in which the cells have fully grown up is counted.

iii). Test Using Yeast (27)

Saccharomyces, and to a lesser extent, *Schizosaccharomyces,* are the yeasts that have most commonly been used in mutagenesis assays. The principal advantage of using such eukaryotic microorganisms is that the assays are relatively simple to conduct and several kinds of chromosome damage can be examined that cannot be detected in bacteria. These assays can be done on a Petri dish, using procedures similar to those described for the *Salmonella* test.

Assays for detection of gene conversion, a chromosomal recombination event, and point mutations at genetic loci where a mutation results in a change in the color of the yeast colonies are often used. Various alterations in the genetic loci controlling the biosynthesis of adenine (a constituent of DNA and RNA) will cause the accumulation of red pigment, resulting in the formation of red colonies. Other changes can block pigment accumulation, resulting in white colonies.

B. Detection of Cytogenetic Effects

Cytogenetic effects of chemicals are usually determined in lymphocytes in peripheral blood, or in erythrocytes in bone marrow. We describe briefly below the three major cytogenetic endpoints that are measured in these assays.

i). Micronuclei

The micronucleus test (28, 29) is based on the observance of extra-nuclear bodies in the cell cytoplasm of red blood cells developing in the bone marrow. Micronuclei in circulating erythrocytes are present at very low frequency (J. MacGregor, personal communication). These bodies originate from either chromosomal breakage fragments or from chromosomes that do not segregate completely during mitosis. Typically, samples of bone marrow are taken at various times after treatment of an animal (usually a mouse) with a test chemical. Bone marrow smears are prepared, and maturing erythrocytes are examined microscopically. Micronuclei are scored in recently enucleated cells that are distinguished from older red blood cells by their staining properties.

ii). Chromosome Aberrations

Chromosome aberrations other than micronuclei can be measured in any body tissue. Chromosome aberrations in peripheral blood are measured in circulating lymphocytes. (30, 31). These are presumed to be exposed to the test chemical either directly, or as they pass through the liver and other organs in which the chemical may be metabolized to active, mutagenic products.

Typically, circulating lymphocytes are collected after treatment of the animal with a test chemical. They are then stimulated to undergo mitosis in culture, which permits the expression of chromosomal abnormalities resulting from DNA lesions produced during the *in vivo* exposure to the test chemical. The cells are appropriately stained, examined microscopically and the various abnormalities are scored. Increased levels of chromosome aberrations in cultured lymphocytes from humans exposed to X-rays and other forms of radiation are well documented (32). Chromosome aberrations in humans resulting from exposure to chemical mutagens have also been reported (33).

iii). Sister Chromatid Exchanges (SCEs)

Sister chromatid exchanges are the result of an exchange of newly replicated DNA and template DNA between sister chromatids at an homologous locus. They can be visualized in metaphase chromosomes by the use of special staining procedures. The molecular mechanism producing SCEs is unknown.

The *in vivo* assay normally involves treating an animal with a test chemical, removing the tissue of interest (often bone marrow or peripheral blood), staining the cells, and examining them for SCEs (34, 35). A variety of mutagens and carcinogens have been shown to induce SCEs in rodents (36, 37), and the assay might be useful as a presumptive test for mutagenic and carcinogenic potential.

iv). Detection of Sperm Abnormalities

A large number of chemical mutagens have been shown to cause an increased incidence of sperm with abnormal morphology when administered to mice (18, 19). Such changes may be caused by genetic effects of the chemical during maturation of the sperm. An higher than normal incidence of abnormal sperm has also been observed in humans exposed to lead (38), and certain drugs (39).

3. Cyclophosphamide: An Example

Cyclophosphamide has been used for many years as an antineoplastic and immunosuppressive drug in the treatment of cancer and some nonneoplastic diseases. It is also a carcinogen, known to cause primarily lymphoreticular and lung tumors in laboratory animals (40), suspected of causing bladder cancers (41, 42) and leukemias (43, 44, 45) in humans.

The anti-neoplastic activity of cyclophosphamide may be due to its ability to cause mutations in the DNA of tumor cells. Cyclophosphamide itself is not mutagenic; reactive chemical species are produced during metabolic transformation of the parent compound.

Plasma (46), urine (46, 47), and bile (10) of laboratory animals treated with cyclophosphamide have been shown to be mutagenic in the *Salmonella* assay. Urine obtained from treated rats produces mitotic gene conversion (48) and point mutations in yeast (49). Patients receiving cyclophosphamide therapy have been shown to have mutagenic urine using *Salmonella* (50), yeast mitotic gene conversion (51), and sister chromatid exchange assays (23). Positive results have also been reported, with urine of nurses dispensing cytostatic drugs, including cyclophosphamide (52).

Cytogenetic effects resulting from exposure to cyclophosphamide have been demonstrated in a variety of tissues in animals and in humans. Chromosome aberrations have been observed in bone marrow (53, 54) and circulating lymphocytes (55, 56, 57) taken from patients treated with cyclophosphamide. Elevated levels of micronuclei in bone marrow (58) and SCEs in lymphocytes (54) are also seen after exposure to the drug. The interpretation of the human studies is complicated by the fact that they must be done in patients who are almost always undergoing multiple drug therapies (56, 58) or a combination of x-ray therapy and chemotherapy (55, 57). Since many chemotherapeutic drugs and x-rays can interact with DNA, it is difficult to be sure that the observed effects were due to cyclophosphamide.

Cytogenetic effects in rodents can be more directly linked to cyclophosphamide treatment because the problems of mixed exposures can be avoided in the laboratory. Cyclophosphamide has been shown to induce micronuclei in rodents (59, 60, 54) at doses within the human therapeutic dose range, chromosome aberrations (61, 62, 63) and SCEs (18) in bone marrow and sperm.

The magnitude of effects produced by cyclophosphamide varies with the species (54) and strain (64) of the animal chosen for study, the route of administration of the test chemical (65), and the timing of the sampling (66). Effects can also vary in different tissues of the same test animal. For example, chromosome aberrations (61) and SCEs (67) are elevated to a greater extent in bone marrow than in sperm. The basis of differences in response in different tissues, or animal species can be due to several factors. These include pharmacodynamic differences in the tissue distribution of the test chemical; differences in the dose required to elicit comparable increases in different genetic endpoints (e.g. it is known that sister chromatid exchanges are induced at lower doses than gross chromosome aberrations); differences between tissues in their abilities to metabolically activate the test chemical to an active mutagenic form; and differences between tissues in ability to repair DNA damage caused by the test chemical.

4. Conclusion

To understand the relationship between mutagenesis, the other endpoints we have discussed above, and carcinogenesis, it will be necessary to design studies capable of identifying common induction mechanisms while taking into account the complexities discussed in the previous section. Toward this eventual goal, we are developing methods for calculating potencies that are quantitative measures of dose-response curves obtained in different short-term tests . We plan to use these to compare results between different tests and between short-term tests and animal cancer tests.

We have developed a procedure for estimating the initial slope of dose-response curves obtained in the *Salmonella* mutagenesis test under the assumption that the initial portion of the curve is linear (68). We are using the estimated initial slope to calculate two alternative measures of potency. These are the 'D5X', the dose of chemical resulting in a 5-fold increase in revertant colonies over the spontaneous revertant background, and the 'D500', the dose of chemical resulting in 500 revertant colonies after subtracting the spontaneous revertant background. Using a large data set obtained from the National Cancer Institute that contains results of multiple *Salmonela* tests conducted using the same protocols in different laboratories, we are comparing these to determine which is the more consistent measure of potency.

We have developed a data-base in which to store the results of these calculations, the dose-response data, and other pertinent information (69). This data-base now contains test results primarily from the published literature and the NCI/NTP *Salmonella* testing program. Data from more than 25,000 dose-response curves from *Salmonella* mutagenicity tests on about 300 chemicals are in the data-base. Data in the data-base and results of the 'D5X' potency calculation are summarized in figure 3A, 3B for the fungicide CAPTAN. The data-base is currently being extended to include results from other short-term tests including mammalian cell mutagenesis, *in vitro* transforrmation, and sister chromatid exchange.

Figure 3. Summary output for *Salmonella* test data including results of the statistical analysis. Figures A and B should be aligned parallel to one another. Each line represents a single dose-response experiment. The columns in Figure 3A refer to pieces of information pertinent to the individual dose/response curves stored in the data-base. Potencies, calculated as the dose to increase the revertant background 5 times, are plotted on a log scale using one of three symbols (+, ±, >) depending on the one-sided *P*-value obtained from the statistical test on the significance of the slope: $+ = (P<.01)$, $\pm = (0.01 \leqslant P < 0.05)$, $> = (P > 0.05)$. Associated lower and upper confidence bounds are plotted as ":". Figure 3B gives detailed bibliographic information about the reference from which the dose/response was taken along with the data themselves. The data are presented as dose/number of histidine[+] revertants pairs. (Adapted from Figure 3 in McCann et. al. (69)).

Figures are on the following two pages.

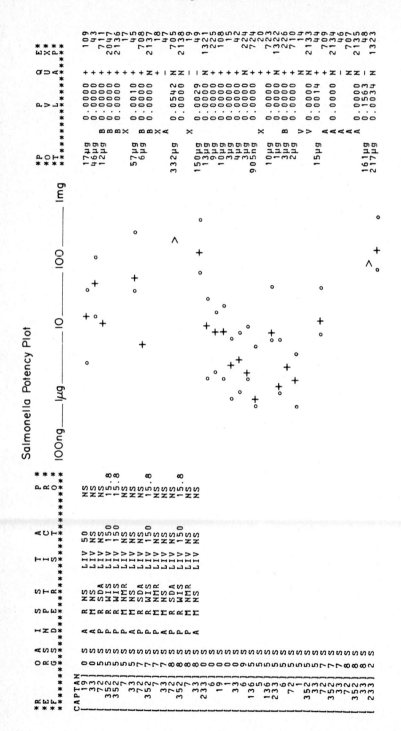

Figure 3A

Mutagens

SALMONELLA POTENCY PLOT   11/18/81

```
CAPTAN
 109 [   19] DeFlora,1978.   NATU,271,p455              0,204,6/ 1,25,223/ 2.5,284/ 5,421/ 10,645/ [5,5]
  43 [   33] Simnon et al.,1977.   EPA,NS               0,(96)/ 1,(141)/ 5,(210)/ 10,(285)/ 15,(340)/ 25,(330)/ 50,(704)/ [7,7]
 711 [   72] Marshall et al.,1976.  JAFC,24,p560        0,14/ 25,117/ 50,231/ [3,3]
2047 [ 3521] Commoner,1976.   EPA,600/1-76-022          0,15/ 13,8,19/ 50,89/ 100,249/ 200,503/ 300,503/ 500,141/ [77]
2136                                                    0,(8)/ 1,(10)/ 10,(15)/ 100,(328)/ [44]
  17 [   71] Herbold, Buselmaier,1976.  MURE,40,p73     [0],[130]/ [1],[129751/ [10],[17.5]/ [20],[0]/ [4]
  45 [   33] Simnon et al.,1977.   EPA,NS               0,(14)/ 1,(20)/ 5,(60)/ 10,(113)/ 15,(55)/ 25,(71)/ 50,(143)/ [7,7]
 708 [   72] Marshall et al.,1976.  JAFC,24,p560        0,9/ 25,148/ 50,288/ [3,3]
2137 [ 3521] Commoner,1976.   EPA,600/1-76-022          0,(10.5)/ 1,(8)/ 10,(7.5)/ 100,(58.5)/ [44]
  18 [   71] Herbold, Buselmaier,1976.  MURE,40,p73     [0],[55]/ [1],[345]/ [10],[0]/ [20],[0]/ [4]
  47 [   33] Simnon et al.,1977.   EPA,NS               0,(3)/ 1,(2)/ 5,(2)/ 10,(2)/ 15,(0)/ 25,(0)/ 50,(1)/ [7]
 705 [   72] Marshall et al.,1976.  JAFC,24,p560        0,32/ 25,32/ 50,51/ [3,3]
2138 [ 3521] Commoner,1976.   EPA,600/1-76-022          0,(11.5)/ 1,(10.5)/ 10,(18)/ 100,(24.5)/ [44]
  19 [   71] Herbold, Buselmaier,1976.  MURE,40,p73     [0],[215]/ [1],[1302.5]/ [10],[26]/ [20],[0]/ [4]
  49 [   33] Simnon et al.,1977.   EPA,NS               0,(25)/ 1,(19)/ 5,(22)/ 10,(26)/ 15,(21)/ 25,(46)/ 50,(44)/ [7,7]
1321                                                    0,224/ 5,2973/ 20,4644/ 50,2593/ [4,3]
 225 [   61] McCann et al.,1975.   PNAS,72,p979         0,154/ 1,302/ 10,972/ 50,1716/ 100,262/ [5,3]
 108 [   19] DeFlora,1978.  NATU,271,p455               0,226,3/ 1,25,325/ 2.5,397/ 5,570/ 10,1115/ [5,5]
  15 [   11] Shirasu et al.,1977.  OHCA,A,p267          0,206/ 1,3,412/ 2,5,882/ 10,2528/ 25,1970/ 50,1118/ [6,4]
  42 [   33] Simnon et al.,1977.   EPA,NS               0,(72)/ 1,(211)/ 5,(532)/ 10,(822)/ 15,(820)/ 25,(720)/ 50,(T)/ [7,3]
 224 [   61] McCann et al.,1975.   PNAS,72,p979         0,27/ 5,282/ 10,349/ 50,211/ [4,3]
 724 [ 1361] Hallett et al.,1975.  Chemical Control     0,5/ 1,6/ 10,10/ 25,18/ 50,67/ 100,84/ 250,2000/ [7,7]
  20 [    5] Seiler,1975.  PCST,17,p398                 [0],[1]/ [9.9E-04],[1.24]/ [0.011],[1.83]/ [0.11],[4.321/ [1],[3.73]/ ***[7]
 723 [ 1361] Hallett et al.,1975.  Chemical Control     0,4/ 1,11/ 10,12/ 25,20/ 50,66/ 100,180/ [6,6]
1322 [ 2331] Ames,1976.                                 0,28/ 5,697/ 20,1722/ 50,366/ [4,3]
 226 [   61] McCann et al.,1975.   PNAS,72,p979         0,16/ 1,35/ 5,106/ 10,163/ 50,275/ [5,3]
 710 [   72] Marshall et al.,1976.  JAFC,24,p560        0,10/ 10,248/ 25,320/ 50,596/ [4,3]
  14 [   11] Shirasu et al.,1977.  OHCA,A,p267          0,NS/ 5,118/ 10,265/ 25,382/ 50,118/ [5]
2133 [ 3521] Commoner,1976.   EPA,600/1-76-022          0,(6,5)/ 1,(13)/ 10,(99)/ 100,(7)/ [44]
  44 [   33] Simnon et al.,1977.   EPA,NS               0,(18)/ 1,(29)/ 5,(80)/ 10,(76)/ 15,(104)/ 25,(80)/ 50,(T)/ [7,5]
 709 [   72] Marshall et al.,1976.  JAFC,24,p560        0,7/ 10,335/ 25,47/ 50,0/ [4]
2134 [ 3521] Commoner,1976.   EPA,600/1-76-022          0,(5.5)/ 1,(4)/ 10,(19)/ 100,(0)/ [44]
  46 [   33] Simnon et al.,1977.   EPA,NS               0,(7)/ 1,(2)/ 5,(5)/ 10,(0)/ 15,(0)/ 25,(0)/ 50,(0)/ [7]
 707 [   72] Marshall et al.,1976.  JAFC,24,p560        0,32/ 10,19/ 25,11/ 50,0/ [4]
2135 [ 3521] Commoner,1976.   EPA,600/1-76-022          0,(7)/ 1,(5)/ 10,(10)/ 100,(10)/ [44]
  48 [   33] Simnon et al.,1977.   EPA,NS               0,(8)/ 1,(7)/ 5,(14)/ 10,(16)/ 15,(26)/ 25,(6)/ 50,(22)/ [7,7]
1323 [ 2331] Ames,1976.                                 0,61/ 5,67/ 20,65/ 50,118/ [4,4]
```

Figure 3B

References

1. Cairns, J., *Cancer:Science and Society,* Freeman, San Francisco 1978, 199 pp.

2. Ames, B. N., Identifying environmental chemicals causing mutations and cancer, *Science,* 204, pp. 587-593, 1979.

3. Hollstein, M., J. McCann, F. A. Angelosanto and W. W. Nichols, Short-term tests for carcinogens and mutagens. *Mutation Research,* 65:133-226, 1979.

4. Legator, M. S., L. Truong and T. H. Connor, Analysis of body fluids including alkylating of macromolecules for detection of mutagenic agents. In: *Chemical Mutagens Principles and Methods for their Detection,* (A. Hollander and F. J. DeSerres eds.) Vol. 5 pp. 1-23, Plenum Press New York.

5. Bruce, W. R., A. J. Varghese, R. Furrer and P. C. Land, A mutagen in the feces of normal humans. *Origins of Cancer,* Book C. pp. 1641-1646, 1977.

6. Lederman, M., R. Van Tassell, S. E. H. West, M. F. Ehrich and T. D. Wilkins, *In vitro* production of human fecal mutagen. *Mutation Research,* 79: 115-124, 1980.

7. Kuhnlein, H. V., and U. Kuhnlein, Mutagens in feces from subjects on controlled formula diets. *Nutrition and Cancer,* Vol. 2: 119-125, 1980.

8. Ehrich, M., J. E. Aswell, R. L. Van Tassell and T. D. Wilkins, A.R.P. Walker, and N. J. Richardson, Mutagens in the feces of 3 South-African populations at different levels of risk for colon cancer. *Mutation Research,* 64: 231-240, 1979.

9. Moriya, M., T. Ohta, F. Sugiyama, T. Miyazawa and Y. Shirasu, Assay for mutagenicity of bile in Sprague-Dawley rats treated subcutaneously with intestinal carcinogens. *J. Natl. Cancer Institute,* Vol. 63: 977-982, 1979.

10. Connor, T. H., G. C. Forti, P. Sitra, and M. S. Legator, Bile as a source of mutagenic metabolites produced *in vivo* and detected by *Salmonella.*

11. Pamukcu, A.M., E. Erturk, S. Yalciner, U. Milli and G. T. Bryan, Carcinogenic and mutagenic activities of milk from cows fed bracken fern (*Pteridium aquilinum*). *Cancer Research*, 38: 1556-1560, 1978.

12. Petrakis, N. L., C. A. Maack, R. E. Lee and Michael Lyon, Mutagenic activity in nipple aspirates of human breast fluid. *Cancer Research*, 40: 188-189, 1980.

13. Montes, G., C. Cuello, G. Gordillo, W. Pelon, W. Johnson and P. Correa, Mutagenic activity of gastric juice. *Cancer Letters*, 7: 307-312, 1979.

14. Ishizawa, M., T. Utsunomiya, N. Kinoshita and H. Endo, Formation of methylnitrosocyanamide from methylguanidine and sodium nitrate in simulated gastric juice and in stomachs of rats: Quantitative estimation by a mutagenicity assay. *J.Natl. Cancer Institute* 62:71-77, 1979.

15. Endo, H., M. Ishizawa, T. Endo, K. Takahashi, T. Utsunomiya, N. Kinoshita, K. Hidaka and T. Baba, A possible process of conversion of food components to gastric carcinogens. *Origins of Cancer Book C*, pp. 1591-1607, 1977.

16. Cerna, M., P. Rossner, K. Angelis, J. Novakova, R. J. Sram, Mutagenicity studies with nitrofurans. III. Mutagenicity testing of nitrofurylacrylic acid in human blood and urine. *Mutation Research*, 77: 13-20, 1980.

17. Cerna, M. and R. J. Sram, Mutagenicity studies with nitrofurans II. Mutagenicity of nitrofurylacrylic acid for *Salmonella typhimurium*. *Mutation Research*, 77: 1-12, 1980.

18. Wyrobek, A. J. and W. R. Bruce, Chemical induction of sperm abnormalities in mice. *Proc. Nat. Acad. Sci. USA.*, Vol. 72: 4425-4429, 1975.

19. Wyrobek, A.J. and W. R. Bruce, The induction of sperm-shape abnormalities in mice and humans. In: *Chemical Mutagens Principles and Methods for their Detection.,* (A Hollander and F. J. DeSerres eds.) Vol. 5: 257-285, Plenum Press New York, 1978.

20. Yamasaki, E. and B.N. Ames, Concentration of mutagens from urine by adsorption with the nonpolar resin XAD-2: Cigarette smokers have mutagenic urine. *Proc. Natl. Acad. Sci. USA*, 74: 3555-3559, 1977.

21. Durston, W. E. and B. N. Ames, A simple method for the detection of mutagens in urine: Studies with the carcinogen 2-acetylaminofluorine. *Proc. Natl. Acad. Sci. USA,* 71: 737-741, 1974.

22. Siebert, D., U. Bayer and H. Marquardt, The application of mitotic gene conversion in *Saccharomyces cerevisiae* in a pattern of four assays, *in vitro* and *in vivo,* for mutagenicity testing. *Mutation Research,* 67: 1455-156, 1979.

23. Guerrero, R. R., D. E. Rounds and T. C. Hall, Bioassay procedure for the detection of mutagenic metabolites in human urine with the use of sister chromatid exchange analysis. *J. Natl. Cancer Institute,* 62: 805-809, 1979.

24. Ames, B. N., J. McCann and E. Yamasaki, Methods for detecting carcinogens and mutagens with the *Salmonella*-mammalian-microsome mutagenicity test. *Mutation Research,* 31: 347-364, (1975).

25. Luria, S. E. and M. Delbruck, Mutations of bacteria from virus resistance. *Genetics,* 28: 491-511, 1943.

26. Green, M. H. L. and W. J. Muriel, Mutagen testing using TRP+ reversion in *Escherichia coli. Mutation Research,* 38: 3-32 (1976).

27. Zimmermann, F. K., Procedures used in the induction of mitotic recombination and mutation in the yeast *Saccharomyces cerevisiae.* In: *Handbook of Mutagenicity Test Procedures.* Kelbey, Legator, Nichols and Ramel (Eds.). Elsevier/North Holland Publishing, N.Y., N.Y., pp. 119-134, (1977).

28. Schmid, W., The micronucleus test. *Mutation Research,* 31: 9-15 (1975).

29. Schmid, W., The micronucleus test for cytogenetic analysis. In: *Chemical Mutagens Principles and Methods for their detection.,* A. Hollander and F. DeSerres (Eds). V1014, pp. 31-55. Plenum Press New York (1976).

30. Evans, H. J. and M. L. O'Riordan, Human peripheral blood lymphocytes for the analysis of chromosome aberrations in mutagen tests. In: *Handbook of Mutagenicity Test Procedures,* Kilbey, Legator, Nichols and Ramel (Eds.) Elsevier/North Holland Publishers New York, NY, 1977.

31. Cohen, M.M. and K. Hirschhorn, Cytogenetic studies in animals. In:*Chemical Mutagens Principles and Methods for their Detection*, A. Hollander and F. DeSerres (Eds.) Vol 2: 515-534. Plenum Press, New York.

32. Evans, H. J., W. M. C. Brown and A. S. McLean (Eds). *Human Radiation Cytogenetics,* North-Holland Publishing Co., Amsterdam (1967).

33. Evans, H. J., Cytological methods for detecting chemical mutagens. In:*Chemical Mutagens Principles and Methods for their Detection*, A. Hollander and F. DeSerres (Eds.), Vol. 4: 1-30, Plenum Press, New York.

34. Allen, J. W. and S. A. Latt, *In vivo* BrdU-33258 Hoechst analysis of DNA replication kinetics and sister chromatid exchange formation in mouse somatic and meiotic cells. *Chromosoma,* 58: 325-340, 1976.

35. Vogel, W. and T. Bauknecht, Differential chromatid staining by *in vivo* treatment as a mutagenicity test system. *Nature,* 260: 448-449, 1976.

36. Nakanishi, Y. and E. L. Schneider, *In vivo* sister- chromatid exchange: A sensitive measure of DNA damage. *Mutation Research,* 60: 329-337, 1979.

37. Bauknecht, T., W. Vogel, U. Bayer and D. Wild, Comparative *in vivo* mutagenicity testing by SCE and micronucleus induction in mouse bone marrow. *Human Genetics,* 35: 299-307, 1977.

38. Lancranjan, I., H. I. Popescu, O. Gavanescu, I. Klepsch, M. Serbanescu, Reproductive ability of workmen occupationally exposed to lead. *Archives Environmental Health,* Vol. 30: 396-401, 1975.

39. Toth, A, Reversible toxic effect of salicylazosulfapyridine on semen quality. *Fertility and Sterility,* Vol. 31: 538-540, 1979.

40. Cyclophosphamide. Chemical and physical data. *IARC,* Vol. 9: 135-156, 1975.

41. Wall, R. L. and K. P. Clausen, Carcinoma of the urinary bladder in patients receiving cyclophosphamide. *New England Journal of Medicine, Vol. 293: 271-273, 1975.*

42. Fairchild, W. V., C. R. Spence, H. D. Solomon and M.P. Gangai. The incidence of bladder cancer after cyclophosphamide therapy. *The Jounal of Urology,* Vol. 122: 163-164, 1979.

43. Portugal, M. A., C. Falkson, K. Stevens and G. Falkson, Acute leukemia as a complication of long-term treatment of advanced breast cancer. *Cancer Treatment Reports,* Vol. 63: 177-181, 1979.

44. Hochberg, M. C. and L. E. Shulman, Acute leukemia following cyclophosphamide therapy for sjogren's syndrome. *The John Hopkins Medical Journal,* 142: 211-214, 1978.

45. Kapadia, S. B. and S. S. Kaplan, Acute myelogenous leukemia following immunosuppressive therapy for rheumatoid arthritis. *Am. J. Clinical Pathology,* 70(2): 301-302, 1978.

46. Suling, W. J., R. R. Struck, C. W. Woolley and W.M. Shannon, Comparative disposition of phosphoramide mustard and other cyclophosphamide metabolites in the mouse using the *Salmonella* mutagenesis assay. *Cancer Treatment Reports,* 62: 1321-1328, 1978.

47. Pak, K., T. Iwasaki, M. Miyakawa and O. Yoshida, The mutagenic activity of anti-cancer drugs and the urine of rats given these drugs. *Urological Research,* 7: 119-124, 1979. 1979.

48. Siebert, D., A new method for testing genetically active metabolites. Urine assay with cyclophosphamide (Endoxan, cytoxan) and *saccharomyces cerevisiae. Mutation Research,* 17: 307-314, 1973.

49. Bauer, C., C. Corsi, c. Leporini, R. Nieri and N Capetola, A mutagenic test in vivo combining the intrasanguineous and urinary assays. *Mutation Research,* 74: 291-302, 1980.

50. Minnich, V., M. E. Smith, D. Thompson and S. Kornfeld, Detection of mutagenic activity in human urine mutant strains of *Salmonella typhimurium. Cancer,* 38: 1253-1258, 1976.

51. Siebert, D. and U. Simon, Cyclophosphamide: Pilot study of genetically active metabolites in the urine of a treated human patient. Induction of mitotic gene conversions in yeast. *Mutation Research,* 19: 65-72, 1973.

52. Falck, K., P. Grohn, M. Sorsa, H. Vainio, E. Heinonen, L. R. Holsti, Mutagenicity in urine of nurses handling cytostatic drugs. *The Lancet,* 1 (8128): 1250-1251, 1979.

53. Neistadt, E. L., M. L. Gershanovich, B. A. Kolygin, B. N. Ogorodnikova, G. A. Fedoreev, E. A. Chekharina, V. A. Filov. Effects of chemotherapy on the lymph node and bone marrow cell chromosomes in patients with Hodskin's disease. *Neoplasma,* 25: 91-95, 1978.

54. Goetz, P., R. J. Sram and J. Dohnalova, Relationship between experimental results in mammals and man. I. Cytogenetic analysis of bone marrow injury induced by a single dose of cyclophosphamide. *Mutation Research,* 31: 247-254, 1975.

55. Morad, M. and M. El Zawahri, Non-random distribution of cyclophosphamide-induced chromosome breaks. *Mutation Research,* 42: 125-130, 1977.

56. Fischer, P., M. Vetterlein, J. Pohl-Ruling and P. Krepler, Cytogenetic Effects of chemotherapy and cranial irradiation on the peripheral blood lymphocytes of children with malignant disease. *Oncology,* 34: 224-228, 1977.

57. Schmid, E. and M. Bauchinger, Comparison of the chromosome damage induced by radiation and cytoxan therapy in lymphocytes of patients with gynecological tumors. *Mutation Research,* 21: 271-274, 1973.

58. Raposa, T., Sister chromatid exchange studies for in vitro and in lymphocytes of leukemic patients under cytostatic therapy. *Mutation Research,* 57: 241-251, 1978.

59. Trzos, R. J., G. L. Petzold, M. N. Brunden and J. A. Swenberg, The evaluation of sixteen carcinogens in the rat using the micronucleus test. *Mutation Research,* 58: 79-86, 1978.

60. Maier, A. and W. Schmid, Ten model mutagens evaluated by the micronucleus test. *Mutation Research,* 40: 325-338, 1976.

61. Miltenburger, H. G., G. Engelhardt and G. Rohrborn, Differential chromosomal damage in Chinese hamster bone- marrow cells and in spermatogonia after mutagenic treatment. *Mutation Research,* 81: 117-122 (1981).

62. Rathenberg, R., Cytogenetic effects of cyclophosphamide on mouse spermatogonia. *Humangenetik,* 29: 135-140 (1975).

63. Datta, P. K. and E. Schleiermacher, The effects of cytoxan on the chromosome of mouse bone marrow. *Mutation Research,* 8: 623-628 (1969).

64. Emerit, I, A. Levy, J. Feingold, Effet chromosomique de la cyclophosphamide chez differentes souches de souris. *Ann. Genet.,* 19(3): 203-206, 1976.

65. Machemer, L. and D. Lorke, Methods of testing mutagenic effects of chemicals on spermatogonia of the Chinese hamster. *Arzneim. Forsch.,* 25: 1889-1896, 1975..

66. Frank, D. W., R. J. Trzos and P. I. Good, A comparison of two methods for evaluating drug-induced chromosome alterations. *Mutation Research,* 56: 311-317, 1978.

67. Allen, J. W., C. F. Shuler and S. A. Latt, Bromodeoxyridine tablet methodology for *in vivo* studies of DNA synthesis. *Somatic Cell Genetics,* 4: 393-405, (1978).

68. Bernstein, L., J. Kaldor, J. McCann and M. C. Pike, An empirical approach to the statistical analysis of mutagenesis data from the *Salmonella* test. *Mutation Research,* in press.

69. McCann, J., L. Horn, G. Litton, J. Kaldor, R. Magaw, L. Bernstein and M. Pike, Short-term tests for carcinogens and mutagens: A data-base designed for comparative, quantitative analysis. In: *Structure Activity Correlation as a Predictive Tool in Toxicology. Fundamentals, Methods, and Applications.,* L. Golberg (Ed). Hemisphere Press, 1981, (in press).

Some General Comments on Nonidentifiability

Peter Clifford
Oxford University

Anyone who has tried to make sense of real data will, sooner or later, have come across the problem of nonidentifiability. Broadly speaking this means that their first explanation of the data is not the only one. The existence of alternative explanations becomes important when decisions have to be made and particularly so when different explanations suggest completely different courses of action. One of the best examples of this dates back to the 1920's. (For a history, see the papers of Newbold (1928) and Bates and Neyman (1952a, 1952b).) The problem is that of explaining the distribution of the number of accidents per driver over a fixed period of time, for London bus drivers. The distribution has a distinctive shape and the hope was that, if this shape could be explained, then decisions could be made which would reduce the number of accidents.

The first explanation which produced a distribution of the right shape is that for each driver there is a constant risk of accident but that this risk varies from driver to driver. It is clear that to reduce the number of accidents, one would not employ drivers whose risk of accident is high i.e. according to this explanation those drivers who have had accidents already.

However this is not the only explanation. Suppose, for example, that all drivers start off equally prone to accidents but that after they have been involved in an accident they become more cautious and progressively so, as the number of accidents increases. It turns out that this is an equally effective way of producing a distribution with the right shape. But this explanation leads to a completely different course of action from that suggested by the first explanation. To reduce accidents we should only employ drivers who have already had accidents, arguing that they are now cautious and therefore safer.

Obviously, as far as making decisions is concerned this is a highly unsatisfactory state of affairs. We conclude that the true explanation is not *identifiable* by means of data which only provide information about the distribution of the number of accidents per driver per fixed period of time. To sort out the two explanations, data of a different type are required. Ideally, a continuous record of the accident history of each driver should be kept so that changes in accident proneness may be monitored. Failing this, identifiability can be achieved by recording for each driver the number of accidents in two successive periods of time (i.e. by mounting some form of longitudinal study of the phenomenon). The moral is that the range of explanations which have to be distinguished should dictate the way in which the phenomenon is observed.

Another more recently studied example of nonidentifiability of particular interest in epidemiological studies of cancer is the problem of determining the effect of eliminating a particular disease from the population. A great deal of data is available, relating to length of life and cause of death in human populations. At first sight, it seems obvious that the effect of removing one disease should be to extend the average lifespan of the population. Furthermore it should be possible to use the available data to estimate the expected increase in lifespan. In order to make the calculations the following analogy has been suggested. The potentially lethal diseases compete in a race. They develop independently, each running its own course at its own speed. The first disease to reach a lethal condition, i.e. to get to the end of the course, is the cause of death and the elapsed time is the lifespan. If this is the true explanation then the effect of removing a disease is to remove a competitor in the race so that on average the time taken to run the race is reduced.

However, once again, the first explanation is not the only one. Tsiatis (1975) showed that it is not possible to determine whether diseases progress independently using data which consist solely of cause of death and life span. Thus in principle it is possible to suppose that the presence of disease A (say measles) either speeds the progress of disease B (say cancer) or slows it down. In general the nature of disease dependence is not identifiable with data of this type. Furthermore the consequence of a certain of action i.e. eliminating a particular disease, may be quite different, depending on whether diseases are cooperative or antagonistic in their interaction, i.e. depending on aspects of the disease process which we cannot identify. Once again longitudinal studies, using comprehensive medical histories can resolve these difficulties. However, such data are very rarely available in human populations and with animal studies there are many practical problems in making relevant observations. Compromises have to be made both in the quality of the observations and in their frequency, and nonidentifiability may be reintroduced by this means. In general problems of nonidentifiability exist all the while there are aspects of any proposed explanation which are not directly observed, but the effect of the nonidentifiability may be quite small. Whether a particular experiment will enable such ambiguity to be reduced to an acceptable level (even with arbitrarily large sample sizes) is a question of vital importance which must be answered prior to experimentation.

References

Bates, G. E. and Neyman J. (1952a). "Contribution to the theory of accident proneness, I. An optimistic model of correlation between light and severe accidents". *Univ. of Calif. Publ. in Stat., Vol. I*, pp 215-254.

Bates, G. E. and Neyman J. (1952b). "Contribution to the theory of accident proneness II. True or false contagion". *Univ. of Calif. Publ. in Stat., Vol. I*, pp 255-276.

Newbold, E. M. (1928) "A contribution to the study of human factors in the causation of accidents". *Indust. Health Res. Board Report No. 34*, London H. M. Stationery Office.

Tsiatis A. (1975) "A nonidentifiability aspect of the problem of competing risks". *Proc. Natl. Acad. of Sci., Vol. 72*, No. 1, pp 20-22.

… PROBABILITY MODELS AND CANCER
L. Le Cam and J. Neyman (editors)
© North-Holland Publishing Company, 1982

The Limits of Nonidentifiability in Time-dependent Compartment Models with Applications to Serial-sacrifice Experiments

Peter Clifford

Oxford University

1. Introduction

This paper is concerned with the very common situation in statistics in which individuals under observation can be in one or another of a finite number of states, the states changing as time goes on. At one extreme the individuals considered may be animals in a carcinogenesis experiment with the states corresponding to a categorisation of current health in terms of diseases present and at the other extreme they could be radioactively labelled molecules injected into a mouse with the states corresponding to possible locations of the molecules in particular organs of the animal.

Without information to the contrary it is usually assumed that individuals behave independently. It is further assumed that changes in state take place according to some random process. What is of interest is the probabilistic rate at which a particular change or transition occurs. This rate will, in general, depend on time, either age with animals or elapsed time following injection in the case of radioactively labelled molecules.

If individual transitions can be observed directly, the estimation problem has a straightforward solution, but typically this is not the case. More commonly it is necessary to infer the transition rates from observations consisting only of the number of individuals in each state at various points in time, that is, without being able to make repeated observations on the same individuals -- either because it is impossible to isolate individuals or because the process of observation is destructive.

There are identifiability problems associated with estimating the time-dependent transition rates. The special case of constant transition rates, i.e. the time-homogeneous compartment model, has recently been investigated by Delforge (1981). For the general case some results are indicated in Clifford (1977) and the effects on statistical analysis are described in Berlin, Brodsky and Clifford (1979). The immediate purpose of this paper is to establish general conditions for identifiability in the time-dependent case and to show how to obtain bounds on the transition rates in the case of nonidentifiability.

2. Mathematical Formulation

Let us denote the state of a randomly chosen individual at time t by $X(t)$ and let $V = \{v_1, v_2, \cdots, v_m\}$ be the set of possible states. Physical considerations will determine whether a transition from one particular state to another is possible. Let $E = \{e_1, e_2, \cdots, e_n\}$ be the set of ordered pairs of states for possible transitions. We assume V and E do not change with time.

Let $P_k(t) = Prob(X(t) = v_k)$ and $P_{jk}(s, t) = Prob(X(t) = v_k | X(s) = v_j)$, $s < t$. Denote the initial distribution by π where the vector π has elements $\pi_k = P_k(0)$. Assume that the process is sufficiently regular that the limit as $\tau \to 0$ of $\tau^{-1} P_{jk}(t, t+\tau)$ exists for $j \neq k$. The limit $\lambda_{jk}(t)$ will be called the transition rate from state v_j to state v_k. The limit exists when, for example, $X(t)$ is a Markov process (in which case $P_{jk}(s, t)$ and $\lambda_{jk}(t)$ do not depend on events earlier than s or t respectively) or when $X(t)$ is obtained by lumping together the states of a Markov process which has a larger and possibly more realistic state space. Suppose, for example, that the v's are symptoms of diseases. It is unrealistic to believe that future health is completely determined by current symptoms or lack of them. It is more reasonable to suppose that the early development of a disease is unrecorded and that symptoms are merely delayed indications of this basic underlying process.

With the regularity conditions the following differential equations can be written down:

$$\frac{dP_k}{dt}(t) = \sum_{j \neq k} \lambda_{jk}(t) P_j(t) - P_k(t) \sum_{j \neq k} \lambda_{kj}(t) \tag{1}$$

where $k = 1, 2, \cdots, m$. So that for a large class of processes, equations of the Kolmogorov forward type are satisfied. It is clear that if π and the λ's are known, the equations can be solved to give the P's. However, if $X(t)$ is not a Markov process, the λ's will depend on the initial distribution π, so that knowledge of the λ's for a particular initial distribution does not enable the P's to be determined for any other initial distribution. Even if π is fixed there are problems in determining $P_{ik}(t, s)$, $i \neq k$. Although similar equations are satisfied,

$$\frac{dP_{ik}}{dt}(t, s) = \sum_{j \neq k} \lambda_{jk}(t, s, i) P_{ij}(t, s)$$
$$- P_{ik}(t, s) \sum_{j \neq k} \lambda_{kj}(t, s, i), \tag{2}$$

the λ's are now, in addition, functions of i and s and are related to known functions only by weak constraints of the form

$$\sum_i \lambda_{jk}(t, i, s) P_i(s) = \lambda_{jk}(t). \tag{3}$$

We cannot determine $\lambda_{jk}(t, s, i)$ from $\lambda_{jk}(t)$ and hence it is impossible to determine $P_{ik}(t, s)$.

For this reason we consider that inference based on transition rates is relevant only if the Markov assumption is made; the λ's then become parameters of interest rather than random variables. From this point we shall make this assumption.

Equation (1) can now be written in matrix from as

$$A D \lambda = b \tag{4}$$

with the following notation. Both b and λ are vectors, b with elements $\frac{d}{dt} P_k(t)$, $k = 1, \cdots, m$ and λ having as its jth element the transition rate corresponding to the jth transition, e_j, at time t. The matrix A has elements a_{ij} given by

$$a_{ij} = -1 \quad \text{if } e_j = (v_i, v_k) \text{ for some k}$$
$$= +1 \quad \text{if } e_j = (v_k, v_i) \text{ for some k}$$
$$= 0 \quad \text{otherwise.}$$

This is the incidence matrix of a directed graph G. The matrix D is diagonal with jth diagonal element given by P_i where i is the subscript of the first element in the transition e_j. Note that both D and b depend on the initial distribution, π, but that with the Markov assumption λ is independent of π. An alternative matrix representation is useful. Let Λ be the $m \times m$ matrix whose off-diagonal elements are $\lambda_{jk}(t)$ and whose diagonal elements are $\lambda_{kk}(t) = -\sum_{j \neq k} \lambda_{kj}(t)$. Then

$$b = \Lambda^T P \tag{5}$$

where P is the vector with elements $P_k(t)$. Let $R = \{P_{jk}(0, t)\}$ then $P = R^T \pi$ so that

$$b = \Lambda^T R^T \pi \tag{6}$$

3. The Likelihood

We assume that individuals behave independently and that each individual can be observed only once. We shall be interested in the case in which the only observations made are the numbers of individuals in particular states.

In certain situations, such as serial-sacrifice experiments, additional independent observations can be made of direct transitions from live to dead states with associated pathology. As has been argued before (Clifford, 1977), in the strict sense, these data do not present problems of identifiability for the rates associated with observed transitions, although, of course, the purely statistical problem of estimation remains. It is therefore possible to reduce the identifiability problem to that associated with a system in which no transitions are observed directly.

The data are thus multinomial and the likelihood of observing an individual in state v_k at time t is simply $P_k(t)$ (which depends implicitly on π). The experimenter may design the experiment by choosing an initial distribution π and an observation time t. In practice the choice of π will be restricted. The dependence of the likelihood on the parameter λ is given in (1).

In general, the likelihood of an observation from a parametric family of distributions will be a function $f(x, \theta, \delta)$ of the observation x ($\epsilon \, \Omega$), the parameter θ ($\epsilon \, \Theta$) and the design δ ($\epsilon \, \Delta$).

Definition: The parameters are nonidentifiable iff for every $\theta \in \Theta$, there exists $\eta \in \Theta$, such that $\eta \neq \theta$ and $f(x, \theta, \delta) = f(x, \eta, \delta)$, for every $x \in \Omega$, $\delta \in \Delta$.

Consider the case where π is fixed and cannot be varied by the experimenter. Assume that the graph G is connected and that π is such that $P_k(t) > 0$ for all k.

Theorem 1: The λ's are nonidentifiable iff G has cycles.

Proof: From graph theory (see for example Bondy and Murty (1976)) recall that a cycle is a path without orientation along the edges of the graph such that the edges are not used twice and such that the starting and ending vertices coincide. Observe that knowing the likelihood for a multinomial sample is equivalent to knowing $\{P_k(t)\}$ and this in turn involves λ via the equation (1). The parameter λ is nonidentifiable if there is another vector μ whose elements are nonnegative such that $\mu \neq \lambda$ and $b = AD\mu$. This is equivalent to the existence of a vector $x \neq 0$ such that $ADx = 0$ since for any such x, provided the elements of λ are positive, there is an ϵ sufficiently close to zero that $\lambda + \epsilon x$ has nonnegative elements. Since the elements of D are nonzero this is equivalent to the existence of $y \neq 0$ such that $Ay = 0$. Now A is an $m \times m$ matrix and since G is connected $n \geq m-1$. But $\sum_i a_{ij} = 0$ for all j so that the rank of A is less than or equal to $m-1$. Suppose that G is a tree (i.e. G contains no cycles), then $n = m-1$. By renumbering the vertices if necessary and omitting the first row, the matrix A can be brought into triangular form with nonzero elements on the diagonal. It follows that the rank of A is $m-1$, so that $Ay = 0$ implies $y = 0$, i.e. if G contains no cycles then λ is identifiable.

Suppose now that G has cycle c. Let E_c be the set of edges of G involved. Choose a direction to go round the cycle. Let y be a vector of length n such that

$$\begin{aligned} y_j &= +1 \quad \text{if } e_j \in E_c \text{ and } e_j \text{ has same direction in } c \\ &= -1 \quad \text{if } e_j \in E_c \text{ and } e_j \text{ has opposite direction in } c \\ &= 0 \quad \text{otherwise.} \end{aligned}$$

It follows that $Ay = 0$, i.e. λ is nonidentifiable, which concludes the proof.

In what follows ideas from graph theory and linear programming are used. The books of Bondy and Murty (1976) and Trustrum (1971) are a good introduction. The space of vectors y such that $Ay = 0$ is called the cycle space of the graph G. It is well known that this space is spanned by the y-vectors associated with cycles. It follows that this space has a basis consisting of such vectors. We shall say that a cycle is directed if the nonzero elements of the y-vector all have the same sign.

In the next theorem we consider the set $N(\lambda)$ of parameters which are indistinguishable from λ, i.e. $N(\lambda) = \{\mu: b = AD\mu, \mu \geq 0\}$.

Theorem 2:
(i) $N(\lambda)$ is convex.
(ii) $N(\lambda)$ is unbounded iff there is a directed cycle in G.

Proof (i) If μ_1 and $\mu_2 \in N(\lambda)$ then $\rho\mu_1 + (1-\rho)\mu_2 \in N(\lambda)$ for all $0 < \rho < 1$.

(ii) Because the elements of D are positive we can equivalently study $\{y: y \geq 0, b = Ay\}$. This convex set has extreme points which correspond to spanning trees of the graph G. The edges of the convex set correspond to basic cycles of the graph. The set is therefore unbounded if there is an edge which is unbounded, i.e. if one of the cycles has a y-vector whose terms all have the same sign.

The set $N(\lambda)$ can be explored by linear programming. The problem of determining the maximum or minimum value of any linear function of the parameter μ subject to the constraint $\mu \in N(\lambda)$ is the standard problem of linear programming for which the simplex method is known to provide a fast numerical solution.

Example

When the graph has few vertices the bounds can be written down explicitly. For example, consider the model for disease development illustrated in Figure 1.

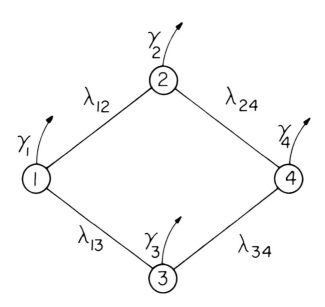

Figure 1. Transistion graph for which explicit bounds of nonidentifiable parameters can be calculated.

There are 4 live states and 4 time-dependent transition rates $\lambda_{12}(t)$, $\lambda_{13}(t)$, $\lambda_{24}(t)$, and $\lambda_{34}(t)$, between live states. In addition, transitions from live to dead states are possible at rates $\gamma_1(t)$, $\gamma_2(t)$, $\gamma_3(t)$ and $\gamma_4(t)$. We shall assume that the γ's are known: $\gamma_1(t) = \gamma_2(t) = 1$, $\gamma_3(t) = 3$, $\gamma_4(t) = 0.5$,

$t > 0$, and that initially the system is in state 1. Suppose now that the true values of the λ's are constant, equal to 1 for all $t > 0$, then solving for the P's we can determine D as follows

$$D = diag\{e^{-3t}, e^{-3t}, e^{-3t}(e^t-1), e^{-3t}(1-e^{-t})\}. \qquad (7)$$

The graph has only one cycle; the associated y-vector is $(1, 1, -1, -1)$. $N(\lambda)$ consists of vectors of the form

$$\mu = \lambda + \epsilon D^{-1} y; \ \mu \geq 0. \qquad (8)$$

It follows that the maximum transition rate from v_3 to v_4 is $1 + (1-e^{-t})^{-1}$ for $t > \log 2$ and $(e^t - e^{-t})/(1 - e^{-t})$ for $0 \leq t \leq \log 2$. The minimum is zero for all t. This is illustrated in Figure 2.

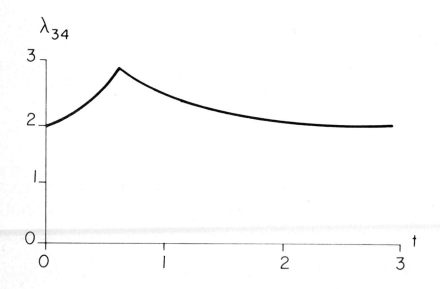

Figure 2. Upper bound for λ_{34} with graph given by figure 1. Lower bound is zero.

Varying the initial distribution

It is clear that when the initial distribution is fixed, severe constraints have to be placed on E in order to have identifiability; the number of nonzero transition rates must be less than the number of states. By observing the P's for a variety of initial distributions considerably more can be achieved. Suppose that k different initial distributions $\pi^{(1)}$, $\pi^{(2)}$, ... , $\pi^{(k)}$ are selected. Denote the matrix with these columns by Π. Then using the representation in (5) we have

$$b^{(i)} = \Lambda^T P^{(i)}, \quad i = 1, 2, \cdots, k \tag{9}$$

so that

$$B = \Lambda^T R^T \Pi \tag{10}$$

where B has columns $b^{(1)}$, $b^{(2)}$, ... , $b^{(k)}$ and superscripts correspond to the initial distributions. If $k = n$ and the matrix Π is nonsingular, then noting that R^{-1} always exists we have $\Lambda^T = B(R^T\Pi)^{-1}$. (i.e. Λ can be determined for a completely arbitrary graph.)

The intermediate case where $1 < k < n$ is more complicated. Identifiability will depend on both the initial distribution and the graph structure. Thus λ is identifiable if the partitioned matrix, whose row blocks are $AD^{(i)}\lambda$, $i = 1, 2, \cdots, k$, has rank $\geqslant n$. In the alternative representation (9), we require that enough constraints be placed on Λ to obtain a unique solution. If we assume that $\pi^{(1)}$, $\pi^{(2)}$, ... , $\pi^{(k)}$ are linearly independent, the equation (9) provides mk constraints on the m^2 elements of Λ. In addition there are m constraints given by

$$\Lambda 1 = 0 \tag{11}$$

where 1 is a vector all of whose elements are 1. These constraints are not linearly independent of (9). Together they place a total of $mk + m - k$ constraints on the elements of Λ. To determine Λ uniquely an additional $m^2 - mk - m + k = (m-1)(m-k)$ constraints are required. The simplest way of doing this is to prohibit certain transitions, i.e. set some of the off-diagonal elements of Λ to zero. Since at least $(m-1)(m-k)$ have to be zero, it follows that the graph G must have no more than $k(m-1)$ edges and we have proved the following:

Theorem 3: If k initial distributions are possible and the graph G has more than $k(m-1)$ edges then the transition rates are nonidentifiable.

However it is not sufficient to reduce the number of edges to $k(m-1)$ because the constraints may be linearly dependent. A constraint of the form $\lambda_{jh}(t) = 0$ is said to be useful if it is among no more than $m-k$ of the form $\lambda_{ih}(t) = 0$, $i \neq h$. It is useful because it is linearly independent of the constraints given by row h of (9). Of course, it may still be dependent on the combination of (9) and (11).

Theorem 4: If k initial distributions are possible and there are less than $(m-1)(m-k)$ useful constraints then the transition rates are nonidentifiable.

Example

To illustrate the use of this theorem consider the two graphs in Figure 3.

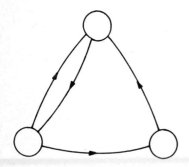 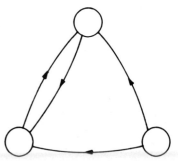

Figure 3. Left-hand graph has identifiable transition rates when 2 independent initial distributions are available whilst the right-hand graph has nonidentifiable transition rates.

Assume that two linearly independent initial distributions are available. Then a direct verification shows that the graph on the left has identifiable transition rates, whereas the one of the right does not. In the latter case we have $m = 3$, $k = 2$ but there are two constraints on transitions into state v_3 and none into the other states, i.e. the total of useful constraints is only one. So that the right hand graph is nonidentifiable by theorem 4.

When there are $(m-1)(m-k)$ useful constraints the question of identifiability reduces to direct verification of the rank of the constraint matrix, i.e. the combination of (9), (11) and the useful constraints. As an illustration consider the graph in Figure 4.

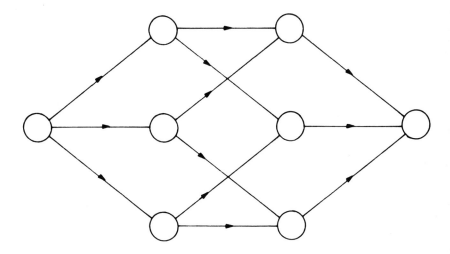

Figure 4. Graph with 8 states and 12 transitions. The transition rates are identifiable if 2 independent initial distributions are available.

There are 12 transitions and 8 states. This is the nonidentifiable component of a model used for 3 progressive diseases, the states corresponding to all disease combinations. The 12 transition rates are nonidentifiable using a single initial distribution but if $k = 2$ the maximum number of identifiable parameters is $(m-1)(m-k)$ or 14. This means that by introducing extra parameters a test of the model with two "degrees of freedom" is possible.

4. Discussion

(i) We have shown that when only one initial distribution is available, the parameters of a time-dependent compartment model are nonidentifiable, unless the underlying transition graph is a tree. However if we are prepared to assume that the rates are constant in time they become identifiable and in principle they can be identified in an arbitrarily brief period of time. It is natural to approximate the time-varying rates by step functions. In this way, one might argue that the parameters should become identifiable in the limit as the step functions approximate the rates. The fallacy in this argument derives from the loose usage of the word identifiable. Although constant rates are identifiable within the class of constant rates, they are nonidentifiable within the class of time-dependent rates. Thus at each stage the step function will have associated a class of indistinguishable time-dependent parameters and this class will persist as the limit is taken.

(ii) The second point concerns the use of the several initial distributions. It might be argued that in experimental radiation carcinogenesis it is possible to alter the initial state of health of the animals by varying the radiation dose. Hence transition rates become identifiable. The problem is that this experimental system provides a severe test of our belief in the Markov hypothesis as far as observable health characteristics are concerned. If animals are sacrificed immediately after irradiation, both treated and untreated animals will appear to be in the same state of health but subsequent developments will show that these initial symptoms were misleading.

Thus although in principle multiple initial distributions resolve the identifiability problem it is necessary to have very strong faith in the Markov assumption i.e. to believe strongly that one is observing aspects of the process which encapsulate all relevant current information.

5. Acknowledgement

This to record my indebtedness to Professor J. Neyman for his help and encouragement over the years. I dedicate this paper to his memory.

Berkeley 1981

6. References

Berlin B., Brodsky J. and Clifford P. (1979) "Testing disease dependence in survival experiments with serial sacrifice" *J. A. S. A.* Vol. 74 No. 365 pp 5-14.

Bondy J. A. and Murty U. S. R. (1976) *Graph Theory with Applications* American Elsevier, New York.

Clifford P. (1977) "Nonidentifiability in stochastic models of illness and death" *Proc. Natl. Acad. Sci.* Vol 74 pp 1338-1340.

Delforge J. (1981) "Necessary and sufficient structural conditions for local identifiability of a system with linear compartments" *Math. Biosciences* Vol 54 pp 159-180.

Trustrum K. (1971) *Linear Programming*, Routledge and Kegan Paul Ltd., London.

Radiation Carcinogenesis - Perspectives

E. J. Ainsworth

Biology and Medicine Division
Lawrence Berkeley Laboratory
Berkeley, California

1. Introduction

When Professor Neyman invited me to participate in this Interdisciplinary Cancer Study Conference and described its objectives, my response was one of considerable enthusiasm because I feel strongly positive about interdisciplinary communications. Next I was presented with the considerable challenge of what to present, and I chose the subject of radiation carcinogenesis more as a student of the subject than a "hands on" expert. I have devoted more than a decade to lifespan studies on rodents where carcinogenesis is the premier endpoint. It is with pleasure that I share my views and experience.

Being aware of the roster of distinguished speakers and the subjects they intended to cover, I felt it would be possible for me to contribute to an interdisciplinary colloquy by presenting first somewhat of a general overview and background information on the problem of radiation carcinogenesis, for the principal benefit of persons in the audience who are nonexperts in this area. I will also attempt to define terminology and describe certain radiobiological phenomena relevant to radiation carcinogenesis. Finally, I will present selected examples of largely new phenomena that, hopefully, will be of interest both to the mathematical modelers and the biologists in this audience. My objectives are to provide perspectives and to call attention to aspects of this problem that persons striving to make important contributions to the study of radiation carcinogenesis through mathematical modeling might wish to consider. My personal opinion is that role of mathematical modeling in this research area is great, because if the question is risk of radiation carcinogenesis at "low doses", estimates of risk for any species, including man, will probably not come directly from empirical data. Estimates will most likely come from mathematical models that benefit from data collected from several species over a range of doses that is higher than the "low dose region", together with careful consideration of both the physics and the biology of radiation carcinogenesis. My principal objective here is to highlight some of the major physical and biological factors of importance.

In organizing the first part of this presentation, I have relied heavily on the report of the National Academy of Sciences committee on Biological Effects of Ionizing Radiations (BEIR Report) (1) and recent overview presentations made to the Director of the National Institutes of Health by Drs. Fry and Burns (2, 3). Since most appropriate references are contained in those documents, and persons interested in obtaining references to original work can consult them, no attempt is made here to cite all appropriate original work in support of general concepts presented. In the second part of the presentation I emphasize selected original work to illustrate certain phenomena I consider important for adding perspective and a dimension of criticality for those interested in radiation carcinogenesis. The research area I know best, life span studies and *in vivo* carcinogenesis, is emphasized.

2. Aspects of the Problem

Carcinogenesis:

Let me first attempt to put the problem in perspective by discussing briefly the carcinogenic process and ionizing radiations. Apologies are expressed to the several experts in the audience whose understanding of these factors exceeds mine! By way of definition, carcinogenesis is a multi-staged process that involves disruption of mechanisms that control cell division, cellular growth, differentiation, and tissue organization. When you studied mitosis in high school or college biology, you were considering the fundamental biological process of cell division and its control. Many aspects of the biology of control systems influencing mitosis, cell population kinetics, and differentiation in normal tissues remain an enigma. It is quite clear that control systems operate ineffectively on cancer cells. The genesis part of carcinogenesis is a particularly intriguing problem that goes well beyond radiation, ionizing, or non-ionizing, and includes other environmental toxicants as well as "spontaneous" alterations in biological control systems.

Realms of Scientific Input:

Because of the nature of the problem, the phenomenon of carcinogenesis has attracted the interest of scientists in many areas. Included here are radiation-oriented scientists as well as others who use viruses or chemicals. Important information also comes from more fundamental studies not concerned directly with carcinogenesis. The physicist is concerned with matters that relate to the deposition of dose at the molecular, cellular, and tissue levels of organization. The molecular biologist strives to understand how cellular machinery, including control machinery, really works through interactions between DNA, RNA, and proteins. Radiation has frequently been used as a tool to produce disruptions in the organization of DNA or DNA/protein in order to understand better this intricate process. Because what a cell, tissue, or organism does is under the direct control of the genes, or DNA sequences of which they are composed, the geneticist is also interested in radiation carcinogenesis. Genetically determined differences in susceptibility to or expression of cancers in various species, including man, have attracted the attention of a significant cadre of mammalian geneticists. Others interested are the physiologist, the radiation biologist, the immunologist, and last, but by no means least, the mathematical modelers and physicians. This assortment of scientific expertise has sought to understand mechanisms of carcinogenesis, provide estimates of risk of radiation carcinogenesis at "low doses" in the occupational exposure range, and promote the treatment or cure of human cancer.

Ionizing radiation is considered to be a "complete carcinogen" in animals in the sense that radiation is capable of both induction and promotion of cancers. It seems useful to introduce here the concept that not all neoplastically transformed cells are ultimately expressed as cancers. Abnormalities termed as preneoplastic lesions or morphologic alterations are seen in some tissues and it appears that these may or may not progress depending upon the complexity of the internal milieu and various host factors that influence tumor expression. Prostatic cancer in man is an excellent example. Much more information is needed to dissociate cancer induction, promotion, and expression as fundamentally distinct and important biological processes. Because I do not plan to consider further the matter of interactions between ionizing radiations and other substances in the environment, I will mention here that the extent to which ionizing radiation may influence the promotion or expression of cancers "induced" by other carcinogens is an area of active thought and investigation. Ionizing radiation has the capacity to, among other things, kill cells and thereby produce perturbations and compensatory mitotic activity in cell populations; induced cell-proliferation could influence the expression of cancer.

Homeostasis: Early Radiation Studies

By way of historical perspective, one of the very early uses of ionizing radiation in animal experiments was to produce cell population perturbations, through cell killing, and study of the processes by which the animal returns to what is known as the "normal steady-state". Homeostasis is the process by which cell populations, dividing or otherwise, and levels of importance metabolize such as sugar or various hormones are maintained at "normal level". The term homeostasis is often used to describe the processes by which normal steady-state conditions are re-established after some type of perturbation such as receipt of a dose of ionizing radiation or ingestion of a large quantity of sugar. Important questions are now being raised regarding the extent to which the normal steady-state is achieved following high doses of ionizing radiation, and the matter of effects of low doses of radiation on maintenance of steady-state conditions is a subject of speculation. Thus, radiation has been used as a tool to study basic mechanisms of cell control and related processes that could influence susceptibility to carcinogenesis and expression of the cancer.

Uses of ionizing radiation, experimentally, have fallen into two general categories: first, the evaluation of homeostasis and the basic mechanisms of cell control, or lack thereof, as indicated by carcinogenesis; and second, the estimation of the risk of various radiation effects in man, including death within 60-120 days from bone marrow failure after high doses delivered over a short period of time. It is well known that radiation biology, as a separate research area, had its origins largely in weapons-related research, the initial objective of which was to provide answers relative to tactical military operations. An example of this would be survival after an atomic explosion where effects of blast and heat are not considered, and the degree of early radiation damage to the dividing cells in the intestine and bone marrow determine survival. risk. Another example is the estimated duration of time troops could function effectively, or survive, when operating in areas contaminated heavily by radioactive fallout from nuclear weapons. These issues were the principal objective of the Manhattan Project and many other studies on external radiations such as X-rays, gamma rays, neutrons of various energies, and radioactive isotopes that may be incorporated into the body through inhalation, ingestion, or puncture wounds. Although it had been appreciated well before World War II that ionizing radiations were carcinogenic in man, it was not until well into the 1950s that fairly large scale experimental studies with rodents were initiated to evaluate specifically the carcinogenic effects of ionizing radiation. In the 1950s significant studies began with both rodent and beagles to asses the carcinogenic effects of both external radiations and radioisotopes.

It was once thought that radiation generally accelerated the aging in animals. At this point and time, we tend to think of ionizing radiation in terms of inducing specific disease processes, such as cancer, rather than an overall acceleration of "natural" aging. Over the decades enthusiasm for large-scale animal experiments to study radiation carcinogenesis has waxed and waned, and although I will return to this matter subsequently, the only point I wish to make here is that because of the extreme complexity of the biological processes that influence transformation of cells from a normal state to a neoplastic state and influence the expression of neoplastic diseases, it is likely that animal experiments will continue to be needed, on some scale, in the future to increase our understanding of the mechanisms of carcinogenesis and the various genetically-controlled "host factors" influencing the expression and natural history of cancer.

3. Physical Factors

Perspectives: Dose-Response Relationships

An important societal concern is the risk of radiation-induced cancer in man. This is patently obvious from what we read in the newspapers, and these concerns may have a huge effect on the ultimate selection of appropriate energy sources for the highly industrialized and wealthy countries of the world. As a practical concern, the fundamental question is the shape of the dose-response curve for cancer in man. It is fair to say that, at this time, human data are inadequate to define accurately the shape of the dose-response curve for any cancer. Consequently, assumptions are made with respect to shapes of dose-response curves where results expressed as absolute or relative risk of cancer induction from studies at "relatively high radiation doses" are interpolated to low radiation doses for radiations of different qualities. According to the most recent BEIR report, the estimates of risk provided are considered to be conservative (1). Let me attempt now to put this matter into somewhat better perspective by re-emphasizing that the principal concern is the carcinogenic effects of low doses, but I will be so bold as to specify that from my point of view, a low dose is below 30 or 50 rem.

Dose Rate Effects

Because most human exposure occurs at low instantaneous dose rates (in terms of rem/minute), the question of dose rate effects is of paramount importance. Cells are endowed with the marvelous capacity to repair radiation injury, including that injury that results in cell death or cancer induction/expression. The greater the time over which a dose of X- or gamma radiation is given, and the lower dose rate the lower is the risk of cell killing, cancer lethality, or life shortening. This generalization applies principally to radiations that are characterized by a low linear energy transfer (LET) such as X- or gamma rays. This generalization does not apply for cell killing and at least for certain cancers when the exposure is to radiations that are characterized by a high rate of linear energy transfer (LET), such as low energy neutrons or alpha particles (1). Also, to the extent that the population considered to be principally at risk for radiation carcinogenesis involves occupationally exposed workers, it is quite evident that exposure to ionizing radiation may occur over a significant fraction of a person's life span. Thus, the effects of radiation experienced at a low dose rate over a significant fraction of the life span is the principal issue. Assessment of risk for occupational exposures requires a fundamental understanding of the effects of repair processes with respect to radiation carcinogenesis, age-related changes in susceptibility to the carcinogenic process, and some understanding of the extent to which perturbations in cell population kinetics in tissues susceptible to carcinogenesis influence either susceptibility to or expression of radiation-induced cancer.

This morning Mr. Neyman presented important ideas with regard to the matter of non-identifiability. It is my belief that assessments of the effects of low dose rate and long exposure times are not understood adequately and the results from animal experiments have been confounded because repair, cell population perturbation and changes related to age-susceptibility to induction and expression are all involved. Very few experiments have been designed or conducted in which the fraction of the life span over which dose is given has been an important feature of the experimental design. I will return to this issue later when I discuss some of the results from experiments with which I have been involved.

Low Dose Rates Fractionation - Repair Processes - LET

In terms of risk assessment and evaluation of fundamental radiobiological responses, the boundary conditions are considered to be represented by low dose rate photon radiation (X- or gamma rays) in comparison with low dose rate neutron or other high LET radiation under circumstances where the fraction of a life span over which doses are given is comparatively long. Viewed in this perspective, occupational exposures are received at low dose rates either on a more or less continuous basis during the workday, or in many isolated episodes that are separated by some radiation-free time. When large blocks of radiation-free time are involved, the exposure is considered to be received in "fractions". Obviously, fraction may also be given at high dose rates. In many cases experimental studies have involved fractionated exposures given at low dose rates over periods of several hours, separated by radiation-free time rather than placing experimental animals in a radiation field where they are exposed continuously for times approaching 24 hours per day. The distinction between more or less continuous exposures and fractionated exposures must be made clear, because in the case of fractionated exposures, the experimental animal is afforded the opportunity to invoke repair processes in the absence of additional radiation injury, whereas, during the course of a continuous exposure, whatever repair processes are invoked must proceed while the radiation exposure is continuing. Repair processes, cell proliferation, and consequently the number of cells at risk for neoplastic transformation could be different for fractionated and continuous exposures. Another complication is that the duration of mitotic (cell division) delay is different for high LET and low LET radiations, and this would be expected to influence the cell population responses after high and low LET radiations, be they delivered at high or low dose rates.

The important point is that "substantive people", to use Professor Neyman's term, performing radiation carcinogenesis experiments have not known the extent to which the effects of doses of gamma radiation administered over approximately 24 hours a day could be "simulated" by the administration of the same daily dose over a period of 8-12 hours a day (at somewhat higher dose rates). Based on a mathematical modeling performed by the late George Sacher and his associates (4), it was thought that the administration of (fractionated) doses of gamma radiation over 8-13 hours per day was an adequate means by which to assess the effects of radiation given over longer exposure times. This was considered to be the case because the slope of the doses response curve was adequately fitted by a slope of 1.0 on a log-log plot where the ordinate was excess mortality rate (from all causes of death) and the abscissa was daily dose rate of gamma radiations. At dose rates in excess of approximately 20-40 gamma rad per day, some recovery processes were invoked, and the dose response curve appeared quadratic, i.e. a slope of 2.0 on the same coordinates. At dose rates below 20-40 rad per day, where the slope of the dose response curve was 1.0, the inference was that no repair or recovery processes could be invoked that would reduce the life-shortening effect of gamma radiation. Thus, it was considered that any further reductions in instantaneous gamma dose rate would have no further effect on life-shortening, excess mortality rate or carcinogenic effects. Emerging data from the JANUS program at Argonne National Laboratory (ANL) have provided new insight into the effects of gamma dose rate and the inferences that may be derived from the Sacher Model (4). It is now clear that at daily dose rates where the slope of the dose-response curve is 1.0, a further reduction in the gamma dose rate permits recovery processes to occur and the effect on life-shortening and incidence of some tumors is reduced.

High Versus Low LET Comparisons

Another important facet of perspective concerns the many comparisons that have been made between high LET and low LET radiations administered over long periods of time. As mentioned above, the least hazardous form of radiation is considered to be gamma radiation, under conditions where the doses have sustained over long periods of time; the most hazardous kind of long-term irradiation is considered to be high LET radiations, from external or internal sources. In radiobiological parlance, such comparisons are designed for assessment of carcinogenic effects where radiations are characterized by two different LETs. The rationale for studies on the LET-dependence of carcinogenesis is that different radiations from both external and internal sources are characterized by different values of LET, and the hazard, in terms of cell killing, mutagenesis, or carcinogenesis is considered to be related to LET. When it is necessary to provide estimates of risk under conditions where a mixture of radiations occurs, and consequently a mixture of LETs, the hazard of each kind of radiation is inferred directly from curves that provide an estimate of quality factor (QF, used for human risk assessment) in relation to LET where QF is estimated from an ensemble of radiobiological data that attempt to define the hazards of radiations characterized by different values of LET. In a sense, the QF is prescribed by committees such as the National Committee for Radiation Protection (NCRP) and they continuously re-evaluate estimates of QF based on emerging results from experiments in which Relative Biological Effectiveness (RBE) has been measured in experimental animals or estimated for humans. RBE is defined as the dose ratio between two radiation qualities, characterized by different values of LET, where the biological effects produced are the same. Thus, where mouse lethality within 30 days from bone marrow failure is the endpoint, the RBE would be 3.0 if the neutron LD50/30 were 300 rad and the LD50/30 for gamma radiation were 900 rad.

RBE-LET Relationship

The concept of RBE-LET relationships is fundamental to radiobiology and radiation risk assessment where carcinogenic and other biological effects are concerned (1). LET is the term used to describe energy *deposition* in relation to a specified path length of the primary radiation or secondary particles. LET is expressed in kilo electron volts (KeV) per micro meter (μm); representative values are of he order of 0.8 KeV/μm for 1.2 MeV gamma radiation from cobalt-60, and of the order of 80 KeV/μm for 0.85 MeV neutrons produced by nuclear fissions in a reactor. In general, the relationship is that the lower (kinetic) energy of the primary radiation, particle or photon, the higher the LET. Thus, neutrons characterized by an energy lower than 0.8 MeV would have a higher value of LET, and neutrons of higher energy would have lower values of LET. Because energy and velocity or wave length are related, an acceptable generalization is that the higher the velocity the lower the energy deposition per unit of path length. The importance of LET, or ionization density in biological systems is related to the magnitude or severity of damage in some volume of the biological target, probably DNA or a DNA-protein complex. One could visualize that many double strand breaks in DNA could be produced by the traversal of a heavy charged particle where the LET is high, and many fewer double strand breaks would result from traversal of a gamma ray where the LET is low and the ionizations produced are separated by, as it were, considerable space. The distinction between LET and dose must be kept in perspective because dose is defined as energy deposited per gram of tissue and does not consider ionization density per unit of path length. Because biological effects are related in some fashion to ionization density, it is evident that a dose of 10 neutron rad would be expected to have very different biological consequences from the dose of 10 gamma rad.

(Dose) Measurements of Dose

Dose to a particular tissue is comparatively easy to estimate for external radiations such as gamma or X-rays or neutrons, but dose is much more difficult to estimate for radioisotopes which enter the body by ingestion, inhalation, or by a puncture wound. In the case of external radiations, tissue-equivalent models are constructed, some anthropomorphic, where the densities of various tissues are considered and ionization chambers or dosimeters of other sorts are placed at different positions within this "phantom". Nevertheless, there are elements of dosimetry associated with external radiations that are quite complicated, such as the estimation or measurement of doses sustained at bone-aqueous (blood) interfaces where bone marrow stem cells (the cells ultimately responsible for production of all blood cells) probably reside, and the doses to cells in bone that are responsible for laying down new bone (osteoblasts). Estimates of dose under these circumstances are obtained by complex calculations that consider all primary and secondary interactions plus the density and locations of the cells at risk. It is evident that if dose to stem cells is an important factor in the induction of leukemia, these considerations are of importance, especially, where estimates are sought for the RBE of weapons neutrons, such as in the populations exposed to atomic bombs in Japan during World War II.

Estimation of dose to specific tissues that result from incorporations of radioisotopes into the body is the subject of many volumes. Both the physical and the biological "half-lives" of the particular radioisotope are considered. The radioactive decay properties of radioisotopes are well known, and assuming that the isotope, such as strontium-90, resides in bone as a substitute for calcium, the time dependent changes in dose rate and total dose accumulated by tissues at risk can be computed. Clearly, if strontium-90 were ingested through milk, the other tissues exposed would be the digestive system and all tissues through which the blood passes before the isotope is finally sequestered in bone. Also, radioisotopes exit the body at a known rate, described by the biological half-life, and other tissues or organs may be irradiated by the presence of radioisotopes in the blood, kidney, and bladder. Obviously, inhaled radioisotopes (radionucleids) involve exposures of the lung. The liver is the site of at least temporary concentration of some radionucleids of interest such as certain plutonium isotopes. Clearly, patterns of dose accumulation in various tissues are quite complicated for radionucleids, and the entire situation is influenced by many physical and biological factors. Also, radionucleids frequently emit radiations of different qualities such as high-LET alpha particles and low-LET electrons or gamma rays providing a very complex radiation field.

Perspectives on Physical Factors in Carcinogenesis

The factors of dose rate effects and LET had been considered above but there are a few additional important points that should be emphasized in order to keep the physical factors involved in radiation carcinogenesis in proper perspective. It is probably fair to say that most critical questions with respect to radiation risk assessment, and revelation of the more basic mechanistic aspects of radiation carcinogenesis, concern the effects of low-LET radiation. Another highly important question is the role of repair processes in reducing carcinogenic risk and/or "fixing the carcinogenic lesions". Although there is general agreement that low-LET radiation administered at low doses over long periods of time is much less hazardous than the same doses administered at high dose rates over short periods of time, such as minutes or hours, the matter of how much hazard reduction or sparing effect for carcinogenesis is a highly contested issue. A recent document published by the National Academy of Sciences, Subcommittee

40, suggests the sparing effect, in comparison with high dose rates, is of the order of 2-10; see (6). This represents a significant departure from previous "conservative" practice where, because the magnitude of sparing effect was difficult to estimate, it had been assumed that the most appropriate approach was to assume no sparing and to accept whatever overestimation of risk would accrue by use of the dose-response relationships inferred from high dose rate experiments.

The matter of dose rate effects for high LET radiations is of considerable interest from both the very basic as well as the applied point of view. It has been appreciated for many years that cellular repair either does not occur or occurs to a much lesser extent after exposure to high LET radiations such as high LET neutrons, and that much less of a sparing effect for radiation carcinogenesis occurs when neutron dose rates are low or fractionated doses of neutrons are administered over significant fractions of the animal's life span (4, 5, 7, 8, 9). Other data emerging from experiments designed to assess more critically the effects of neutron dose rate and fractionation suggest that over some range or doses administered to mice, the carcinogenic, and perhaps other effects of fractionated neutron doses may indeed be greater than the effects of the single dose (8). This will be considered in some detail subsequently.

With respect to the effects of LET, relationships between LET and RBE for cell killing have been described and are currently under investigation in various laboratories where mammalian cells cultured *in vitro* are the endpoint (10). More recent data concern the effects of LET on various proliferative and non-proliferative cells in animals (11). Suffice it to say that for many *in vitro* systems the peak RBE for cell killing occurs at a LET of the order of 100-150 μm, but some recent data on *in vivo* systems such as the mouse testes and intestinal crypt stem cells indicate that peak RBE occurs at a lower LET value (12). Human lymphocytes show a peak RBE for cell killing well below 100 KeV/μm (13), so it is clear that LET-RBE effects differ for different biological systems. The LET dependence of radiation carcinogenesis in mammalian systems has been studied over only a limited LET range primarily with neutrons. Emerging results from both *in vitro* systems about which Dr. Yang will speak later in this conference, and from *in vivo* systems suggest that RBE-LET relationships for neoplastic transformation *in vitro* and carcinogenesis *in vitro* are not yet completely defined.

4. Biological Factors

Genetics

A myriad of biological factors influence radiation carcinogenesis and the interpretation of results from various biological systems as they relate to evaluation of mechanisms as well as providing estimates of radiation risk for man (14). The point to make first is that the biological factors influencing radiation carcinogenesis are of the greatest interest in terms of unravelling mechanisms, and are of the greatest complexity and challenge because of the truly multi-dimensional nature of the problem. As stated above, everything a cell does, or has a capacity to do, is determined totally by its genetic endowment. The complete array of genes in any organism is referred to as the genome, and although the genome of a muscle cell is the same as the genome of a brain cell, during the course of differentiation certain genes and their products have been expressed and others have not because these cells are different structurally and functionally. Different genes or gene products are expressed in different cells in the body of any multi-cellular organism, and in addition to functional differences, those cells may have wholly different radiation sensitivities, capacities for repair of radiation damage, susceptibilities to neoplastic transformation, and responsiveness to various factors in the milieu that influence cell proliferation.

Sensitivity Differences

It is well known that the stem cells of the blood-forming system, (hematopoietic stem cells) in man or mouse are appreciably more sensitive to the lethal effects of ionizing radiations than are the stem cells in the intestine, and the rate of killing per unit radiation dose may differ by a factor approaching 2.0. Likewise, within a particular mouse genotype, where the genes are 99.5% the same among individuals, the capacity to repair radiation injury differs appreciably for bone marrow and intestinal stem cells. It is likely that the differences in radiation sensitivity and repair capacity within a species approximate those between species. Within a genetically homogenous species, different cell populations exhibit marked differences with respect to the fraction of stem cells normally in mitosis (in the cell division cycle), the amount of time required to complete the mitosis, and in the case of tissues like the gut or bone marrow, the total duration of time lapsing between mitosis and the production of a mature functional daughter cell. In bacteria, the genotype determines rigorously all the biochemical machinery of the cell that influences radiation sensitivity, repair capacity, pathogenecity, and the tendency toward mutability. In the much more complex mammalian situation, the animal's genotype determines its life span, tumor prevalence at various ages, cell population kinetics, susceptibility to either bacterial or viral infection, and the influence of radiation in terms of either production of bone marrow, intestinal, or central nervous system, death after doses ranging from a few hundred to several thousand rad. Also genetically determined is susceptibility to radiation-induced life shortening mediated by cancer. One objective of all science is to seek unifying hypotheses that permit certain genotypic factors to be "factored out". It is probably fair to say that, with exceptions of life span or longevity, and radiation-induced life shortening, the availability data in mammalian species are not now sufficient to provide convincing quantitative handles on the effects of mouse genotype on dose-response relationships for carcinogenesis. At the moment I would submit that if one of the "substantive people" presents compelling data on dose-response relationships for tumor x in the zzz strain of mouse, that is exactly what we know. It is not clear now the extent to which we can extrapolate quantitatively or interpolate to other mouse strains or other species. Encouraging results in this area have been presented by Fry (2) and are summarized later in this presentation.

Life Span Studies: Interspecies Comparisons

The life span study represents one experimental approach in radiation carcinogenesis. Doses selected are sufficiently low to avoid death within days or weeks and permit expression of late effects such as cancer. Autopsies are performed on animals found dead or sacrificed when considered in a terminal state. Histopathology is done frequently, and tumor diagnoses are based on the composite autopsy findings; when possible, a most probable cause of death is assigned. The late pathology (distinct from tumors), such as degenerative diseases, infection or hemorrhage, is also recorded. Thus, in addition to tumor incidence or prevalence, mortality data are collected. Mortality data are expressed in terms of mean number of days lost, percent life span shortening (in comparison with unirradiated controls) or age specific death rates. Using mortality data, dose-response curves are constructed and inferences may be drawn regarding effects of dose rate, radiation quality, age at the time of irradiation, sex or species. At any given dose, not all deaths are attributable to a single tumor type, and multiple tumor types are often present (15). Consequently, precise information on specific tumor responses to radiation is not provided by life shortening statistics. However, certain generalities regarding carcinogenesis are possible. For example, if reducing the dose rate from 10 rad/min to 0.01 rad/min had no effect on mortality statistics, a reasonable inference would be that no sparing effect of low dose rate prevailed on the tumor types responsible for mortality. Definition of the extent to which shapes of dose response curves for life shortening portend of dose-response curves for even certain tumor types remains to be established.

With respect to inter-species comparisons, one of the important contributions of the late George A. Sacher was to attempt to provide a unifying hypothesis with respect to life-span shortening among several wild rodent species exposed to gamma radiation doses for the duration of their life commencing at young adulthood (4). Over a certain level of daily dose rates, Sacher found that among rodent species, and possibly in the beagle, a linear dose-response relationship could be inferred, whereas at higher dose rates, the shape of the dose response curve was probably quadratic, indicating the importance of repair/recovery processes. Assuming that these are adequate handles, we now have a means by which to understand certain fundamental radiobiological processes among different species, and we have the hope of obtaining quantitative handles on the degree to which the genome influences these processes. In a similar fashion, Grahn has considered carefully age-specific mortality patterns of mice and man in unirradiated populations, and has suggested that certain transpositions of rodent data to human experience are possible if differences in life span are taken into account (14). These issues are not trivial when one bears in mind that the rationale for most of the animal experiments conducted to evaluate carcinogenic effects of ionizing radiations are expected to contribute to human risk estimation. My opinion is that the data remain inadequate, and more research is necessary before both the virtues and limitations of the extrapolation of the animal data on life shortening or tumors can be assessed critically. It should be noted, parenthetically, that because there is currently no means by which to assess quantitatively the genetic effects of ionizing radiation in man, the mutational studies conducted in mice are extrapolated directly and quantitatively (1).

The basis for species differences in susceptibility to an expression of cancer constitutes a fundamental challenge to our understanding of radiation carcinogenesis. The role played by hormones or other substances that influence cellular proliferation or metabolic activity requires further study to determine their roles in susceptibility to an expression of cancer. Hormone-dependent tumors in animals and man, such as breast and prostate, are well known. Another biological factor that must be considered is the role played by oncogenic viruses that are indigenous to many mouse strains and are known to play some role in the development of cancer such as thymic lymphoma in certain highly susceptible mouse strains, such as the $C57/BL_6$ mouse. Thymic lymphoma is an excellent model with which to illustrate the complexity of radiation carcinogenesis experiments in which this tumor is one of the endpoints, because expression of the disease requires irradiation of at least some portion of the bone marrow and release of an oncogenic virus. Oncogenic viruses in mice are "vertically transmitted" from the mother to the developing offspring as if they were part of the inherent genetic constitution of the animal. Many other viruses in mouse populations have been described, some of which are vertically transmitted and some of which are horizontally transmitted (from one animal to another), and the role played by viruses not considered to be primarily oncogenic in the susceptibility to or expression of cancer is not understood. Among the "substantive people" are those who feel strongly that, although mouse cancers are important to study for the fundamental purpose of evaluating aspects of susceptibility to an expression of radiation-induced cancer, the differences between cancers among various species, including man, are such that great caution must be used in the making of either qualitative or quantitative extrapolations from rodent to other species.

A final example of the extent of which "biological factors" influence carcinogenesis is the myeloid leukemia model in the RF strain of mice that has been studied extensively by Upton and his associates (16, 17). myeloid leukemia is a well known lethal disease in man but occurs at low frequency in many mouse strains. The frequency in most mouse strains, irradiated or unirradiated was sufficiently low so as to preclude this tumor as a model system for studies of radiation-induced myeloid leukemia in man. Due to the genetic constitution of the RF mouse plus other "biological factors", it appeared that this strain might be a suitable model for myeloid leukemia. The initial studies involved experimental animals that were housed "conventionally" and were exposed to the normal assortment of bacteria and viruses that occur in an animal colony where special health precautions are not taken (16). The frequency of myeloid leukemia in unirradiated and irradiated animals appeared sufficiently promising that larger studies were conducted to establish dose-response relationships. Because the ambient bacteria and viral flora were recognized as potentially uncontrollable biological factors that could complicate long term studies, procedures were instituted whereby the bacterial and viral flora were controlled by presenting germ-free mice with a specified microbial flora and attempting to maintain this flora by housing the animals under strictly controlled environmental conditions referred to as maintaining them behind a "barrier". The barrier-maintained animals showed a much reduced frequency of either spontaneous or radiation-induced myeloid leukemia, indicating the complicating role played by the microbial flora in susceptibility to or expression of this disease in either irradiated or unirradiated animals (17). Walburg conducted various interesting and important studies in which the susceptibility of germ free, barrier-maintained, and conventional animals to myeloid leukemia was compared (18). Although "genetic drift" -- that is, small changes in the genetic constitution of the animals as a function of time, a process that normally occurs in all mice -- was not precluded totally as a factor in the experiments on RF mice, the bacterial or viral flora is thought to play the paramount role by influencing the cell kinetics in bone marrow.

Finally, multi-cellular organisms, including mammals, are endowed with a highly complex immune system which mounts responses to "foreign substances" such as viruses, bacteria, or the presence of foreign mammalian cells within the body such as skin or bone marrow transplants. Animal's immune system has a remarkable capacity to identify "foreign" from "self" based the chemical structure of proteins or protein complexes, referred to as antigens that are present. The good news is that the immune system plays an important role in combatting various infectious diseases, and the bad news is the immune system is involved in allergic responses and "autoimmune diseases" of which rheumatoid arthritis is probably an adequate example. Antigenic changes have been reported in cancer cells in experimental animals and man, immune substances have been detected in the blood of affected hosts, but the role played by the immune system in the expression of the neoplastic diseases is not understood fully. The integrity of the immune system in mammals and its capacity to respond to antigenic changes in cancer cells, is another biological factor that must be considered in radiation carcinogenesis.

To recapitulate briefly, all aspects of the cellular sensitivity to ionizing radiation, including capacity to be transformed and express this alteration are all under genetic control. It is generally accepted that DNA or DNA protein complexes are the target of ionizing radiations and that repair or misrepair plays an important role to fixation of radiation-induced lesions by cell proliferation. Different cells within a species are known to differ with respect to their radiation sensitivities, repair capacities and tendencies for neoplasia. Significant differences exist with respect to the capacity of transformed cells in various tissues to be expressed as tumors and this also occurs between species. The biology of tumor expression, or latent period, is quite complex and must be explored much further. In fact, in many tissues, the size of the (stem) cell population at risk for radiation carcinogenesis is not known. Also, perhaps cells other than stem cells are at risk as well.

5. Experimental Radiation Carcinogenesis Approaches

Early in this presentation I mentioned the various scientific disciplines within the realm of biology and other research areas where contributions to radiation carcinogenesis were being made. Now I would like to specify several different realms within the broad context of biology where important research is underway and will help understand the mechanisms of carcinogenesis and assist with the matter of prediction of human risk. These various fields are largely complementary, yet each has its limitations as well as advantages.

Molecular Biology

The importance of the genome in all biological processes has already been stressed. The study of molecular biology strives to understand genes, their chemical structure, how nucleotides and bases are linked, how disordering affects gene products, and how various chemical or physical agents disrupt genes and all their products. Within the realm of molecular genetics are studies that are concerned with fundamental aspects of mutagenesis, and prokaryotic organisms such as viruses or bacteria are largely used for these studies. The "substantive people" who do research in this area have selected these organisms based on their comparatively simple genetic constitution because the number of genes or gene products is very small in comparison with the number that would occur in a mammalian cell. In certain organisms such as *Escherichia coli* elaborate genetic maps are available so that the location of various genes or their subunits are described completely in the transcriptional sequence on the bacterial chromosome. Fundamental important new contributions have been made in terms of understanding DNA replication, factors that control it, the synthesis and control of various gene products, and how various chemical and physical agents disrupt this fundamental biological process. Our understanding of genes and their alterations through mutation have come largely from work with prokaryotic systems.

The capacity of microorganisms to mutate has been described carefully for several decades, and more recently Professor Ames has developed methods whereby forward and reverse mutations in *Salmonella typhimurium* (the organism which causes the mouse's version of typhoid fever) can be measured accurately after exposure to various chemicals or physical agents (19). Relationships between mutagenesis and neoplastic transformation are not understood. However, many feel that mutagens are also carcinogens, and identification of substances that produce mutations in bacterial or mammalian cells are at least candidates for careful consideration in terms of the carcinogenic potential (20). Through the use of the methodologies pioneered by Prof. Ames, it is clear that important new contributions to our understanding of mutagenesis and the basis for that process will occur, and those results probably also have some relevance to the question of the carcinogenecity of various agents in more complex (eukaryotic) biological systems. However, the challenge remains with regard to how to extrapolate or interpolate information gained regarding mutagenic effects in prokaryotic systems to eukariotic systems, let alone the question of the relationships between mutagenesis and transformation in mammalian cells. Much remains to be learned regarding the *in vivo* relevance of dose-response relationships for mutagenesis measured in prokaryotic systems. My feeling is that the principal contribution from studies on prokaryotic systems will be in terms of unravelling mechanisms of mutagenesis and repair of DNA damage that result in mutation. At this point and time we are not clever enough to know how to utilize such elegant data fully to predict mutagenic or transformational events in mammalian cells and certainly not clever enough to be able to predict how data obtained using prokaryotic systems can be used qualitatively for human risk assessment.

Mammalian Cells Cultured in vitro

Since Puck and Marcus first described procedures whereby mammalian cells could be cultured *in vitro* very much like bacterial cells, an extensive body of radiobiological information has accumulated, and many fundamental contributions to our understanding of radiationbiology had been made (21, 22). Because mammalian cells cultured *in vitro* are handled very similarly to bacterial cells, many of the same physical and biochemical probes used in the study of prokaryotic systems have found application in mammalian cells, such as the measurement of DNA damage. Many cell lines have been established from various animal species and humans, and it must be recognized that, by definition, mammalian cells that proliferate on artificial media are not presented with the same cellular or humoral growth control factors that are present in the tissues or organs from which they originated. Often cell lines propagated *in vitro* have abnormal numbers of chromosomes, in comparison to cells in the tissue or origin, and it is probably fair to say that adversaries are quick to point out that many of the cell lines propagated *in vitro*, and studied extensively, had many "abnormal" characteristics. This is not necessarily meant as a criticism, and only as a means by which to add perspective to use of biological generalizations or specific data attained in experiments with mammalian cells cultivated *in vitro*. For example, it is known that several radiation responses, including cell killing and mutation, differ between various established cell lines and between cell lines and primary explants; primary explants are "recently" isolated cells, primarily fibroblastic, that have been passaged for weeks or months, rather than years or decades as is the case for cell lines. Their degree of "normality" not withstanding, our understanding of the dose-response relationships for cell killing, the effects of repair on both cell killing, mutagenesis transformation, and the effects of LET on these processes, and the relationship between these processes and DNA alterations has come largely through studies on cells propagated *in vitro* (23, 24). Again, as with prokaryotic systems, we are not clever enough now to utilize these results to predict quantitatively the radiobiological responses of cells *in vivo* where they are subject to many of the "biological factors" specified above. The extent to which data obtained on cell killing, repair, mutation, or transformation can be extrapolated or interpolated to the intact mammal, including man, remains to be elucidated. Perspective on interpretation of data on *in vitro* transformation is honed by the recent report that removal of the hormone thyroxin from culture medium eliminates radiation-induced transformation (25). Although the supplies necessary to perform *in vitro* radiobiological studies have increased in cost dramatically over the last several years, this approach to studies of radiation carcinogenesis has been pursued enthusiastically because the cost is minuscule in comparison with the cost of performing large scale life span experiments.

Life Span Studies on Animals

Carcinogenesis studies in experimental animals had been the traditional means whereby the risk of cancer and life-shortening effects of ionizing radiation had been studied. Arbitrarily I will separate the animal studies into two broad categories: namely (1), life span studies and (2), studies with specific tumor model systems. By way of perspective, I will state first that animal studies are quite expensive for reasons that will become obvious, and important questions are raised regarding the extent to which results from mice have applicability to the human experience. Studies on radiation carcinogenesis *in vivo* using mice, rats, rabbits, guinea pigs, or beagles offer the advantage that the expression of the carcinogenic process is studied where the cells at risk, whichever and however many there are, exist in the biological milieu where all of the "biological factors" specified above may come into play. However, the extent to which the liver, lung, or skin tumor in the mouse serves as an adequate model system for human tumors is a popular area for debate. Because of concerns and limitations in extrapolation of animal data to the human experience, less expensive means have been selected whereby the fundamental aspects of carcinogenesis and factors affecting tumor expression can be studied in mammalian systems. Thus, during the last decade, research dollars allocated to animal experiments have dwindled and the emphasis has been placed on *in vitro* studies. As mentioned above, both have their virtues and limitations, and it is not clear that the information sought concerning human dose-response relationships, under a variety of experimental conditions, can be obtained exclusively through data generated by *in vitro* studies of carcinogenesis.

Dating to the days of the Manhattan Project, the life-span study has been the traditional mans by which radiation carcinogenesis *in vitro* has been studied. Many life-span studies had been conducted during the ensuing three decades, and it is fair to say that what we understand about the importance of biological and physical factors *viz.* genotype, dose rate, radiation quality, sex, and age, has come largely from these studies. Few who perform mouse experiments feel that the effects of dose rate or LET would be the same in mouse, dog, and man in any quantitative sense. However, most substantive people who perform such experiments do believe that if reduced dose rate results in a reduced carcinogenic risk in several strains of mice, rabbits, guinea pigs, and dogs, the same qualitative process will occur in man. Unknown at this time is the extent to which qualitative generalization inferred from, for example, dose rate studies in animals can be extrapolated to man in any even quasi-quantitative sense. The question asked is, if four different strains of mice, guinea pigs and dogs, show a 2-5 fold reduction in the frequency of mammary tumors when the dose rate is "low" in comparison with administration of that dose at a "high" rate, is it reasonable to assume that the response of humans would be similar? Only now, are data becoming available to deal rigorously with questions such as this (2). In addition fundamental question about inter-species extrapolations on a quantitative basis, the matter of relationships between lifetime spontaneous rate and radiation-induced cancer rates must also be considered. Fry has recently dealt with this issue and Table 1 summarizes results he has evaluated for various cancers in three mouse strains and in man. The results are interpreted to indicate that the rate of induction (assuming linear dose-response relationships for lifetime incidences) is

Table 1

Natural Incidence/Susceptibility and Radiation Induced Incidence in Mouse and Man

Data From R. J. M. Fry, Proceedings of the Public Meeting
March 10-11, 1980 To Address a Proposed
Federal Research Agenda
Vol. I, pp. 111-136

Tumor Type	Strain	Nat. Incid. (%)	Increased Incid./rad (%)
Ovarian	RFM	2.4	0.39
	Balb/c	6.4	1.2
Mammary	Balb/c	7.5	0.07
Gland	B_6CF_1	1.2	0.01
Myeloid	RFM	4.0	0.14
Leukemia	RFM	3.0	0.09
Chronic			
Gran. Leukemia	MAN	-	1.4-3.6
Myel. Leukemia	RFM	-	3.5
Acute Leukemia	MAN	-	0.6-1.5
Acute Thymic Lymphoma	RFM	-	1.4

influenced by the natural incidents, thus favoring the use of relative risk rather than absolute risk (1). For two types of leukemia, the relative increase in incidence per rad appears to be in the same realm for mouse and man. Whereas no one would debate that acute or chronic leukemias in mouse and man differ in certain properties, it would be indeed encouraging if, within certain cancer "categories", the use of relative risk estimates permits us to surmount the "species barrier", and to better utilize data from experimental animals to predict human cancer responses.

Methods of analysis of tumor data from animal experiments have improved vastly during the last decade. Competing risks are considered in all current data sets, but some care must be taken in evaluation of the earlier data. Attention to the matter of competing risk is attributable, within the radiobiological community, to the efforts of Hoel and Walburg (26). This indicates the desirability of a close relationship between the substantive person who performs experiments on radiation carcinogenesis, and the statistician. If, indeed, life-span experiments are to continue into the future, an important purpose would be served by more careful inter-disciplinary, and inter-laboratory, consideration of experimental design, methods of data collection, and their analysis. I also feel strongly that data collected from life-span experiments should be published in a form such that they can be analyzed critically by all interested scientists. Fry has urged that such practices be instituted (personal communication). This seems wholly appropriate to make full use of data collected from life-span experiments where many millions of dollars have been expended, together with time of the order of at least one decade in the life-span of the substantive people who perform the experiments. Realistically speaking, a decade is not a vast overestimate of the time between planning of a large scale study and the publication of the results in the reviewed scientific literature.

Tumor Model Systems in Animals

Another experimental approach in radiation carcinogenesis has involved the use of specific tumor model systems where the animals are often not maintained on experimental status for the duration of their lives. This cost-cutting procedure and overall approach has its obvious advantages as well as limitations. Specific tumor models such as skin, mammary gland, Harderian gland and to a more limited extent, myeloid leukemia in the CBA mouse, have been used to evaluate the importance of various physical as well as biological factors in radiation carcinogenesis (27-30). In the case of skin, mammary, and in some cases Harderian gland models, only the organ or tissue in which carcinogenesis is to be evaluated are irradiated. This involves either shielding the remainder of the animal or focusing a radiation beam on the target tissue. In a very complete sense, one is dealing with an irradiated target tissue in a normal unirradiated host animal. It is also possible to modify certain biological factors, such as the circulating levels of hormones, in order to address specific scientific questions as they relate to particular "host factors" (28, 29). The duration of time, after irradiation, that animals are maintained on experimental status often depends on the latent period of the tumor, and the limiting condition is whatever duration permits expression of the tumor at the lowest radiation dose used in the experimental design. Mammary and Harderian tumors are hormone-dependent and their latent periods are fairly well known. The latent period for skin tumors has also been described, and the question of importance concerns the relationship between latent period and radiation dose (27). This question is one that benefits from frequent debate. The mammary tumor in the Sprague Dawley rat has been studied extensively and will serve to illustrate a few points of importance. By 12 months of age, unirradiated animals show a significance prevalence of this tumor, and radiation increases that prevalence in relation to radiation dose (28). A question sometimes raised with this tumor model system is the extent to which radiation is acting only as a promoter, or if the radiation damage serves both to induce and promote tumors. Because of the local nature of the irradiation and the fact that potentially lethal mammary tumors may be removed surgically, the population of test animals at risk is not culled by other radiation-induced malignancies or by the induction of a lethal mammary tumor. Although, Harderian gland tumors are not surgically removed, the sacrifice time at which prevalence is determined -- 350-400 days after irradiation -- is sufficiently early so as to virtually preclude a significant numbers of deaths from other causes, including natural "mortality" from tumors or other causes. This means that the competing risk issue is of little importance, and high dollar cost-effectiveness may be touted. The Harderian tumor model system involves tumor promotion by the presence of an excess of steroid hormones, and under these conditions, most tumors are expressed within 350-400 days (29). The CBA leukemia model utilized most extensively by Major and Mole appears to offer considerable potential as a model system under circumstances where hormonal control of influences is not considered to be a major factor (30). Because leukemia in the Japanese population exposed in World War II is of importance and has received particular notoriety, considerable enthusiasm exist for further development and exploitation of a specific model system in mammals for leukemia. Naturally, the cautionary flag concerns the extent to which inter-species differences exist in bone marrow (stem cell) cell population kinetics and how this could influence estimation of susceptibility to leukemia induction and shapes of dose-response curves. In view of the results summarized above, and with respect to relative risks of leukemia in the RF mouse and humans, it would seem particularly important to pursue further studies on radiation leukemogenesis for comparative purposes.

By way of further perspective, it is not clear at this time the extent to which animal studies, either life-span or those utilizing tumor model systems will elucidate either mechanisms of carcinogenesis or provide means by which to estimate carcinogenic risk at radiation doses below 25 rem; namely, those in the occupational realm. As in man, radiation-induced tumors that are clearly "radiation-induced", rather than "spontaneous", are difficult to demonstrate in experimental animals giving low radiation doses at low dose rates over a long period of time. If the fundamental issue for radiation risk assessment is the shapes of dose-response curves for various tumors in man over a range of "low doses", it is not patently obvious, at least to me, that that information will come, in a convincing fashion, from animal experiments. Rather, the likelihood is high that an important contribution to this problem will be made by a combination of fundamental studies involving prokaryotic systems where DNA damage and repair are evaluated, where similar and other processes are studied in mammalian cells cultivated *in vitro*, and fundamental information on mechanisms is viewed critically in the context of results available from animal experiments. Mathematical models that benefit from an appreciation of the complexity of the carcinogenic process *in vitro* and *in vitro* are the only means by which radiation risk at low doses can be estimated meaningfully.

Human Epidemiological Studies

National committees whose onerous charge is to provide *quantitative* estimates of carcinogenic risk for man utilize extensively, if not exclusively, data obtained from epidemiological studies on exposed human populations (1). In a larger sense, this is wholly appropriate, because the biological specimen of interest is man, and a full appreciation of how host factors differ between species, as they relate to induction and expression o radiation-induced tumors, is not fully at hand. The various human population studies are described fully in the latest version of the BEIR report, so suffice it to say here that, as with many animal experiments, those substantive people who deal directly with human populations are confronted with the challenge of extrapolation or interpolation of results obtained at "comparatively high doses" into the low dose region of interest. Where populations of humans have been exposed to ionizing radiation in the low dose range (at low dose rates over significant periods of time), significant carcinogenic effects have not been established unequivocally. It is clear that epidemiological studies on human populations must continue and it is hoped that these efforts will contribute significantly to human risk assessment in dealing directly with societal concern regarding radiation hazards. My personal view is that a definitive answer to the question of carcinogenic effects of radiation at low doses in man, on a quantitative basis, will not come from epidemiological studies alone. I wish to make clear that I have no hesitancy about the adequacy of human data, from both external radiations and internal emitters, for empirical curve fitting over a high range of radiation doses, but as with animal studies, a combination of mathematical models supported by an appreciation of mechanisms in phenomenology will be the means by which human risk at low doses continue to be estimated.

6. Relevant Research on Experimental Animals

Having now dealt with various aspects of background information that I hope will provide perspective to this inter-disciplinary audience, I will now attempt to stimulate the interest, and hopefully the contribution, of the statisticians in the audience in terms of providing mathematical models for emerging phenomenology that is either directly or indirectly related to the fundamental problem of radiation carcinogenesis.

7. Large Scale Animal Studies: Oak Ridge and Argonne National Laboratories

Oak Ridge and Argonne have conducted extensive life-span studies for nearly two decades for purposes of comparing carcinogenic and life-shortening effects of high LET neutrons and low LET gamma radiation. Both the physical and biological factors specified above had been elucidated through these projects. Fig. 1 illustrates 3 putative radiobiological responses where effects of high and low LET radiations are compared. The upper left panel illustrates cell survival after single doses (administered at high dose rates), and the survival curve for high LET radiations is more or less exponential, whereas the low LET survival curve exhibits a "shoulder", and the initial slope(s) and final exponential slope differ. The RBE for cell killing is dependent on total dose. The upper right panel illustrates the putative dose-response relationships for cell-neoplastic transformation *in vivo* or *in vitro* where responses are expected to be linear or quadratic, respectively. One expectation might be that following high LET radiation, the linear dose-response would prevail, whereas, after single doses of low LET radiation, the transformation response might be expected to be more or less quadratic, or linear-quadratic where the quadratic response

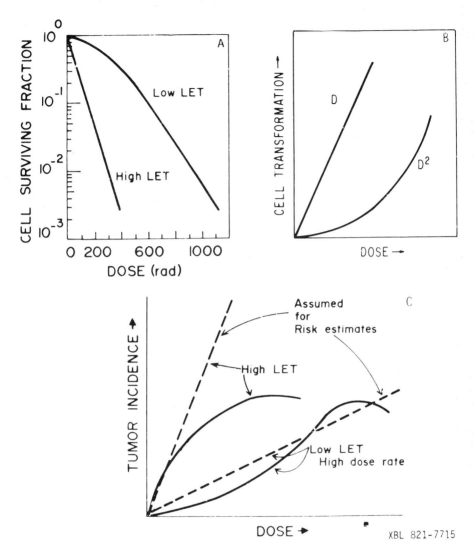

Fig. 1. Generalized representation of responses to high and low LET radiations. (A) Cell survival; (B) assumed relationships for induction of malignant transformation; (C) relationships for incidence of tumors *in vivo* as a function of dose. >From R.J.M. Fry, 1977, reference 59, reprinted with permission.

predominates. Clearly, at low levels of dose on the quadratic curve, it would be difficult to differentiate rigorously, based on curve fitting, between a linear and quadratic dose-response relationship. Again, the RBE for cell transformation would be dose-dependent. The lower panel in Fig. 1 illustrates that currently, for the purpose of risk estimation, bodies charged with that responsibility assume linear dose-response relationships for either single doses administered at high rates or protracted doses administered at low rates, but the slopes for the low and high LET curves differ appreciably. Also shown in the lower panel are nonlinear curves for high and low LET radiation, respectively, that are based on tumor or life-shortening results from several large-scale animal experiments conducted at Oak Ridge or Argonne National Laboratories.

8. Methods and Aspects of Experimental Design

Experimental design and other aspects of the Oak Ridge and Argonne experiments should be appreciated (5, 8, 9, 31, 32). Such matters influence interpretation of results. The objective of both projects was to evaluate RBE in relation to dose and dose rate for carcinogenic effects of radiation; information on life shortening comes free and is the first to be collected. Different mouse strains were used in the two projects where each strain exhibits its own characteristics life-span and tumor expression characteristics. The neutron radiation sources were different. Fission neutrons from 252-Cf were used at Oak Ridge, and fission neutrons from the JANUS reactor were used at Argonne; the neutron, energy spectra and dose-averaged mean LET values probably also differed. At Oak Ridge several mice were irradiated simultaneously within a home cage, whereas at Argonne, mice were irradiated individually in disposable plastic cups. Because several mice were irradiated simultaneously in the Oak Ridge experiments, estimation of the average dose to an individual mouse and the neutron and gamma[1] dose, respectively, experienced by an individual

---

1) Gamma rays are produced within an animal when a neutron is captured; total dose to the animals consists of contribution by both neutrons and gamma rays.

mouse requires careful scrutiny. Dosimetric challenges exist in the Argonne experiments because substantially different estimates of dose are provided assuming that the animal remains on all four feet during most of the exposure or if indeed the animal spends a significant portion standing on hind feet attempting to escape from the plastic cup!

Dosimetric considerations not withstanding, important aspects of he experimental design, as they relate to low rate exposures, also exist between the two projects. Incremental doses of neutrons or gamma radiation in the Oak Ridge experiments were administered by exposing the animals at a more or less constant dose rate for *different* periods of time; that is, low doses were given by exposing the animals for a few days, whereas the larger doses involved exposures of several months. In contrast, the Argonne experiments utilized the design in which instantaneous dose rates *differed* and the total irradiation time (the number of hours the mice were actually being irradiated) was held constant. Also the total fraction of the life-span over which the dose was administered represented one of he experimental variables. Because age at the time mice or rats receive a single (high) radiation exposure influences life-shortening and carcinogenic effects, some attempt has been made to assess age-dependent differences in susceptibility or expression of carcinogenesis or life-shortening (8, 33, 34). Not absolutely clear at this time is the extent to which differences in mouse strain, in experimental design between the two laboratories and different "physical factors" involved in the experiments contribute to differences in experimental results on shapes of dose response curves and effects of dose protraction. These differences are presented here in order to inject perspective, for either statisticians or biologists who might have interest in evaluating, comparatively, results from the Oak Ridge and Argonne experiments.

Because of my role in the design, execution, evaluation, and publication of early results in the Argonne experiments, plus my familiarity with the current status of that project, results from Argonne will be emphasised in making points I hope will be interesting to both the statisticians and biologists.

My interest in the biology of aging, engendered by Professor Herman Chase during my graduate student days at Brown University, plus my interest and experience with high LET neutron radiation, was the basis for my acceptance of the invitation to join the staff in the Biology and Medicine Division at Argonne National Laboratory in 1969. I had the extremely good fortune to be associated with the late George A. Sacher, Douglas Grahn, and R. J. M. Fry in studies of the carcinogenic and other late effects of gamma radiation or neutron radiation from the recently modified JANUS reactor sited in the Biology and Medicine Division. My first assignment from Dr. Grahn, then the Group Leader of the JANUS Project, was to review all of the available literature on carcinogenesis/life-span studies and to provide recommendations with regard to an experimental design that had a high likelihood of providing significant new information, and avoiding the problem of "nonidentifiability". Critical review of the literature indicated: (1) that dose-response relationships for cancers in mice were not established clearly after exposure to high or low LET radiations, administered either at high or low dose rates; however it was clear that some appreciable sparing effect resulted when gamma radiation was given at low dose rates over long periods of time; (2) that marked sex differences were noted in carcinogenic and life-shortening responses, but RBEs for neither carcinogenesis nor life-shortening were defined clearly; (3) that relationships between either single or protracted doses of neutron or gamma radiation were probably linear where the endpoint was excess mortality rate, as stated by Grahn (35), but uncertainties about curve shapes existed; (4) that estimates of carcinogenic and life-shortening effects per unit dose appeared to be influenced by the fraction of a life-span over which the dose was given, but no clear pattern emerged because the experiments were not designed specifically to test hypotheses regarding dose-duration of exposure-relationships; (5) that sensitivity to at least the life-shortening effects of high single doses administered at high dose rates was influenced by age of exposure in such a fashion that life-shortening effects per rad diminished with increasing age, but the role played by this phenomenon in chronic exposure experiments was not clear; both age related changes in sensitivity to carcinogenic effects and factors influencing cancer expression could be involved; (6) that unclear also was the extent to which mouse genotype, control life-span, and the spectrum of tumors that occur in either unirradiated or irradiated animals could play a significant role in the development of predictive models that could assist in the understanding of mechanisms of radiation carcinogenesis *in vivo*, or in the development of predictive models that could be of value in predicting low dose effects and RBE for high LET radiations in man.

Janus Project Experimental Design

The principal elements of the experimental design are illustrated in Fig. 2. The objective was to define dose-response relationships and to assess how carcinogenic/life-shortening responses varied when doses were protracted over 23 or 59 weeks or for the duration of the animals' life. The principal commitment made was to define dose-response relationships for carcinogenesis and life-shortening (a normal fall-out from life-span experiments) after single doses of gamma rays or fission neutrons, and under circumstances where doses were given in fractions, at comparatively low dose rates, over a total duration of 23 weeks. The administration of 24 fractions over the duration of 23 weeks, approximately 25% of he average life-span for unirradiated controls, was selected arbitrarily. It was felt that 25% of the life-span was a significant fraction, and hopefully, would be an adequate representation of the extent to which dose per fraction affected carcinogenic and life-shortening responses. Frankly, cost and logistic challenges were also a consideration, because large numbers of mice were involved in the experiments, the radiation facilities had a limited capacity, and simply performing the exposures was a non-trivial problem based on the personnel available for the project. For all experimental groups with which I will deal, the total exposure time was the equivalent of 45 minutes per fraction for 24 fractions administered over a duration of 23 weeks; thus, all fractionated doses were administered in a total time of 18 hours. In comparison with the effects of single doses administered in a constant exposure time of 20 minutes, fractionation produced a 54-fold increase in exposure time and a variable change in instantaneous dose rate for the

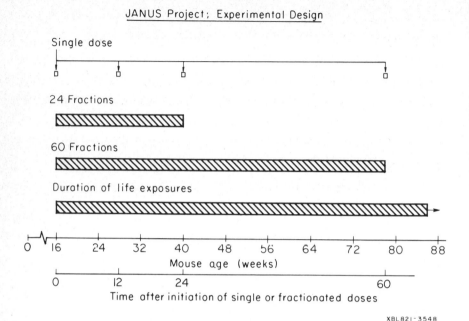

Fig. 2. Schematic representation of the experimental design for Janus project experiments initiated between 1971 and 1975. The mean life span for unirradiated $B6CF_1$ on mice was estimated to be approximately 107 weeks following shown irradiation at 16 ± 1 wk. The rationale was to administer weekly fractionated doses, at low fission neutron or gamma dose rates, over approximately 25% or 50% of the remaining life span, or for the duration of the animal's life. Changes in sensitivity to life shortening and carcinogenic effects of single doses, given at higher dose rates, was to be estimated at four ages.

various dose groups. Sample sizes were large and ranged from of the order of 800 unirradiated controls to of the order of 400/sex/dose at low radiation doses and to of the order of 100/sex/dose at high radiation doses. More limited efforts and reduced sample sizes were devoted to questions of the extent to which protracting radiation doses over fractions of a life-span longer than 25% influences estimates of radiation carcinogenesis in life-shortening. The two additional exposure periods investigated were 59 weeks (approximately half the average life-span of unirradiated control), and exposures for duration-of-life. We wanted to compare carcinogenic effects when the same dose was protracted over either 23 or 59 weeks. To give the same physical dose in 60 fractions over 59 weeks as were administered in 24 fractions over 23 weeks, the weekly exposure time was kept constant at 45 minutes, but the instantaneous dose rate was reduced by a factor of 2.5. Note should be taken here that we have a confounded variable in the 23 vs. 59 week comparison because *both* instantaneous dose rate and the fraction of the life-span over which dose is given differ. To provide for another direct comparison with effects of doses given over 23 or 59 weeks and with earlier duration-of-life results published by Sacher and Grahn (36), two dose groups of animals were irradiated weekly for the duration of their lives using the same instantaneous dose rates and exposure times as were used for the groups that received 60 exposures over 59 weeks. This permitted assessment of the effect of incremental dose received after 59 weeks. Age-related differences in sensitivity to single radiation doses were determined by administering graded doses at approximately 110 days of age (corresponding to the age at which fractionated exposures were initiated), at approximately 190 days of age (corresponding to the approximate mid-point of the 23 week radiation period), and at approximately 270 days (corresponding to the animal's age at the time the administration of 24 fractionated exposures was completed). Additionally, some single doses were given to animals at approximately 520 days of age, corresponding to the animals' age at the time 60 fractions were completed when protracted over 59 weeks.

Insofar as the fractionated doses of gamma radiation are concerned, it is important to point out that the Sacher model (4), and inferences derived therefrom, contributed significantly to the gamma dose selection, and ultimately the selection of fractionated neutron doses. Based on excess mortality rate, results from the Sacher model indicated that, at daily doses of below 20-40 R/day administered over approximately 8-13 hours, the curve relating excess mortality rate to daily dose rate could be adequately fitted (on a log-log plot) by a linear function. Such zero order kinetics imply the absence of repair/recovery and a total-dose dependence for the life-shortening (and possible carcinogenic?) effect over the range of doses explored. An important objective of the JANUS experiments was to evaluate RBE for carcinogenic and life-shortening effects after "low doses", and the linear relationship for gamma radiation, plus the presumed linear relationship for fractionated doses of neutron radiation, provided a rational means by which to estimate, confidently, RBE over a dose range of interest. A constant RBE of 10 was assumed for most neutron doses. This rationale appeared appropriate based upon the "state of the art" at the time the experiments were designed, between 1969 and 1972. The relationship to the Sacher model is important to stress here, because certain aspects of that model are not supported by life-shortening data that have been published recently, as will be described subsequently.

A total sample of the order of 20,000 mice was dedicated to the experiments described above, excluding animals that were given single doses of radiation at ages in excess of 110 days of age. Histopathology has been and is being done on the majority of those animals to establish causes of death, in so far as that is possible, and to diagnose accurately cancers and other diseases observed in that test population. Large amounts of time and effort are required to perform autopsies, collect tissue samples, embed these samples for preparation of microscopic slides, and allow for the evaluation of those slides by a pathologist. Appreciating this, it becomes quite evident why mortality data are analyzed and published well in advance of the time that pathology data, including data concerning tumor dose-response relationships, are presented. A considerable volume of tumor data have appeared in the open literature based on results from the Oak Ridge experiments (31, 32, 37, 38, 39 40), but the assessment of pathology data from the JANUS experiments remains to be completed.

Comments about mortality data from these experiments are appropriate. Data reduction was in terms of excess mortality rates, percent of life-shortening, or days of life-span lost. These are derivatives of average life-span of the test population, in comparison with a control or sham irradiated population. In using average values, "fine structure", which perhaps indicates a large fraction of deaths early in the life-span as the results of a specific disease, is averaged out. Age specific mortality rates, from specific neoplastic diseases, will probably be used more extensively in the future to assess, quantitatively, carcinogenic effects of ionizing radiations.

Only limited inferences can be drawn regarding carcinogenic effects when life-shortening data are presented in the form of some derivative of the averaged survival time. An obvious example of this is the conclusion that, if the life-shortening effects of high and low dose rates were similar, the same inference would hold for the predominant lethal tumor. The converse would be true, for some lethal diseases if a large sparring effect on life-shortening were observed. Histopathology and determination of the most likely cause of death is necessary to establish clear relationships between life-shortening and cancer induction.

Janus Project Results

With the benefit of these caveats I will deal with life-shortening data recently published from the JANUS experiments to illustrate selective phenomena which are considered, by me at least, to be important in the field of radiation carcinogenesis. The early neutron work by Upton and associates indicated that neither dose per fraction nor administration of dose at low dose rates produce a sparing effect on the life-shortening or the incidence of some tumors (37, 38). One of the hypotheses tested in the JANUS experiment was that neutron dose protraction over 23 or 59 weeks of the animals' life span would produce no reduction of tumorigenesis/life shortening in comparison to the effects of the same total physical dose administered to young adult animals at high dose rates. The rationale related to the virtual absence of repair/recovery processes for neutron-induced radiation injury that results in cell killing or neoplasia. In contrast, because repair processes are clearly operational for radiation injury produced by low LET photons, sparring effects were expected, but their magnitude remained a matter of controversy. Life shortening results (Fig. 3) indicate that certain aspects of the hypotheses on which the JANUS experiments were based are not supported for either neutron or gamma radiation. Based on life shortening, over a neutron-dose range of 20-240 rad, a single linear function appears not to be an adequate fit to the data. Other curve-

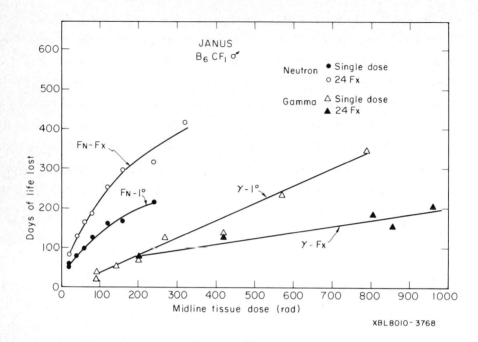

Fig. 3. Days of life span lost in B6CF$_1$ mice given single (1 degree) or fractionated (Fx) doses of fission-spectrum neutrons from the Janus reactor or ^{60}Cobalt gamma radiation. The single or first fractionated dose was given at 110±10 days of age. A total of 24 fractionated doses were given over approximately 24 weeks at low dose rates. Consult Thomson et al. 1981, reference 5, for details of sample sizes, dose rates, and the original data.

fittings, such as two linear curves with different slopes, may provide equally acceptable alternatives to the function used here. The curve is not linear, as expected from earlier work (35), and on the ever popular log-log plot, excess mortality rates for both sexes are characterized by a slope of the order of 0.6, which departs from the expected slope of 1.0 that characterizes certain dose-response relationships for neutrons over at least a selected dose range, such as stamen hair mutations in *Tradescantia* (41).

Fig. 3 also shows that the number of days of lost increased significantly over the dose range of 20-240 rad when the total neutron dose was administered in 24 fractions over 23 weeks rather than as a single dose. The "enhancement effect" is statistically significant in male mice, but not among females, at a total dose of 20 rad where the "low" fractionated doses of 0.83 rad were administered at a "low" dose rate of 0.185 rad/min. The extent to which this enhancement phenomenon obtains in male mice at doses below 20 rad is currently under study under the direction of Dr. John F. Thomson, the current Group Leader for the JANUS project.

A sex difference is apparent and may be greater for neutron than for gamma radiation. Females show a higher sensitivity to the life-shortening effects of neutrons than do males, but this sex difference is less apparent among mice that receive single doses of gamma radiation where the slope on the log-log plot is in the range of 1.2-1.3. Clearly, among the gamma irradiated mice of this strain, the quadratic component does not appear to play a dominant role over the 90-700 rad range. (Fig. 3)

A statistically significant reduction in days of life span lost occurs when gamma radiation doses are administered in 24 fractions over 23 weeks (Fig. 3) when the total doses to males are greater than 417 rad. At total gamma radiation doses of 206 or 417 rad, the number of days of life span lost in males was quite similar after single or fractionated gamma doses. This raises interesting questions with respect to "dose rate effects" on those neoplastic diseases, in this strain of mouse, that account for life-shortening at low doses and low levels of life shortening. When Thomson used a linear regression model to fit days of life span lost versus radiation dose for animals that received either acute or protracted gamma ray doses, the linear coefficient for animals given fractionated exposures was approximately half that for animals given singular exposures when the dose range considered was from 206-1110 rad (5). Thus, the sparing effect of protracted gamma radiation is estimated at approximately 2 and effects could be greater at higher doses, and less or absent at doses of 417 and 206 rad in male mice.

Other interesting results concern the extent to which the estimate of days of life span lost is influenced by the fraction of the life span over which protracted doses are given. Comparisons involved protracting neutron or gamma doses over 23 or 59 weeks or for the duration of the animal's life. The first comparison I will consider involved reducing the weekly dose rate and increasing the number of fractions and duration of exposure from 24 fractions in 23 weeks to 60 fractions in 59 weeks. Table 2 and Fig. 3 show the number of days of life lost when neutrons were administered in 60 fractions totalling 40 or 160 rad, fall interestingly close to the values obtained when animals were exposed to 24 fractions. Thus, *reduction* of the neutron dose per fraction and instantaneous dose rate, together with an *increase* in the duration of exposure to 59 weeks, produce no reduction in life-shortening. In contrast a reduction of life shortening was observed when comparable circumstances prevailed for gamma-irradiated mice.

The comparison between 24 and 60 fractions is clearly an invitation to further work with both neutron and gamma radiations. Accepted at face value, the results indicate several interesting departures from current thinking. Beyond the fact that the results indicate that the RBE is higher for 60 fractions than for 24 fractions, and that neutron-dose per fraction and dose-rate exhibit total-dose-dependent properties, whereas gamma radiation does not, fundamental questions can be raised about the LET-dependence of tumor induction/expression, assuming the life shortening at these doses is attributable to tumors. By definition, the production of radiation injury ceased at 23 and 59 weeks, respectively, after initiation of the radiation exposures. Because the life shortening response among neutron animals is the same, it is clear that the dose "integrates" fully and important changes in *susceptibility to* neutron-induced life shortening do not occur. The neutron results with 24 and 60 fractions indicate clearly that the life span remaining to the irradiated animals is fully adequate for expression of the latent period of whatever tumors cause the animals' demise. The similarity of life shortening when neutron exposures were given over 23 or 59 weeks is particularly interesting. Assuming that the causes of death are the same in the two populations, questions are raised about the biological factors that influence expression of the disease processes that cause the animals' demise. Why is the life shortening the same when the period of exposure differed by nearly 6 months? Were tumor latent periods different under these exposure circumstances? What are the factors that influence tumor progression independent of the number of transformed cells. Hopeful results on tumor frequencies/pathology in these groups will shed light on these issues.

In the case of gamma radiation administered at low dose rates in 24 and 60 fractions, we have a confounded variable (non-identifiability?) where discrimination between repair of tumorigenic injury and availability of sufficient after-expectation of life for tumor expression are confounded. Again the weekly doses per fraction and instantaneous dose rates were decreased by a factor approaching 2.5 while the number of fractions was increased from 24 to 60. This resulted in a significance reduction of the number of days of life span lost. This may mean that it is the radiation injury produced relatively early in the animal's life span which is expressed most fully. This may also point to the matter of age-related alterations in susceptibility to radiation-induced neoplasta and life shortening. Here again inherent susceptibility and time for expression may be inextricably confounded. Results from a pilot experiment presented years ago indicated the possibility of LET-dependent differences in susceptibility to or expression of life shortening injury after single doses of neutron or gamma radiation (8); it will be important to see if replicate experiments now in progress yield similar results.

By way of added perspective, it must be borne in mind that the relationship between age-related changes and susceptibility to or expression of radiation injury produced by single doses administered at high dose rates fail to provide a means by which to establish how susceptibility or expression changes during the course of a protracted irradiation episode. Clearly, in one case one is measuring the response of "normal" steady state systems, and in the other case, various steady-state systems have been perturbed, the cell population kinetics are different, and the role of these perturbations in susceptibility or expression is not understood.

As mentioned above, definition of the "susceptible fraction of lifespan" has plagued all who have attempted to design experiments where protracted irradiation has been used. When duration-of-life exposures are given, most would agree that the last rad received on the day of death probably has not contributed to induction (and possibly not even to expression) of the life shortening disease. Results of Neary *et al.* (42) and Upton (38) raised important questions about the susceptible period and the matter of "wasted radiation". Although any incremental radiation dose could influence tumor expression, and the same could be said for various other environmental factors, including chemicals or microorganisms that influence cell population kinetics, definition of the dose that induces and permits expression of a (lethal) neoplastic disease is not readily determined by experiments designed for duration of life exposure. The data available are very limited, but results from the JANUS experiments permit comparison of life shortening, and ultimately tumorigenesis, when fractionated radiation doses were given over 60 weeks, or under circumstances where that same weekly dose is continued for duration of life (Table 2). The essential point is that incremental doses received after 60 weeks -- that is, following approximately one half of the animal's normal average expectation of survival -- contributed very little to life shortening. It should be noted that in several instances the incremental dose amounted to several hundred rad; under these circumstances dose is expressed at the mean accumulated dose to the test population. Thomson *et. al.* have reported no differences in life span when either neutron or gamma doses were given in weekly fractions over 60 weeks as compared with duration of life (9); consequently, the results have been pooled and comparisons have been made with results from duration of life experiments reported by Grahn and Sacher where the gamma radiation doses were given 8-13 hours per day for duration of life. Based on days of life span lost per weekly fraction/rad, it is estimated that the fractionated doses administered in 45 minutes per week from the JANUS experiments were approximately twice as effective as were the fractionated exposures used by Grahn and Sacher where the exposure times were longer and the exposures were given 7 days/week. This means that repair/recovery processes are operative at low instantaneous dose rates for gamma radiation. It might be speculated further that

Table II

Life Span Shortening in B$_6$CF$_1$ Mice Given Fractionated Doses of Fission Neutron or Gamma Radiation in 24 or 60 Fractions or for Duration of Life (DOL). From J. F. Thomson et. al., Radiat. Res. 86, 573, 1981 and ibid. 86, 559, 1981.

Dose/Fraction (rad)	No. Fractions	Males		Females	
		Mean Accumulated Dose (rad)	Life Shortening (Days) ± SE	Mean Accumulated Dose (rad)	Life Shortening (Days) ± SE
Fission Neutrons					
1.67	24	40	129±17	--	--
0.67	60	40	111±18	40	88±39
0.67	DOL	74	123±17	DOL	115±15
2.67	60	160	267±15	160	252±13
2.67	DOL	244	259±20	211	298±33
Gamma Radiation					
17.4	24	417	126±17	417	107±19
7	60	417	37±18	417	66±42
7	DOL	813	80±16	813	32±15
80	24	1918	487±19	--	231±13
32	60	1918	274±15	1918	231±13
32	DOL	2888	266±17	2750	249±38

were the weekly gamma doses for 7 days per week and 24 hours per day, the life shortening/carcinogenic effects would be reduced further. If the term "chronic irradiation" is defined as exposures administered 24 hours/day, the ensemble of results indicates that weekly fractions given at low dose rates (less than 1 rad/minute) are not an adequate surrogate for truly chronic exposures because of the operation of the repair processes for gamma radiation. However, in the case of neutrons, the available data indicate that because of the absence of repair processes, weekly fractions given at dose rates less than 1 rad/minute probably represents an adequate surrogate for radiation doses administered at even lower dose rates over 24 hours/day. Thus, in the context of the Sacher model, the existence of a linear dose-response curve over a range of low weekly doses *does not* preclude the operation of repair processes that serve to diminish carcinogenic and life shortening effects of gamma radiation (4). Also, the enhancement phenomenon for neutrons was not considered in the Sacher model because the data were not available at that time. The existence of zero order kinetics for description of excess mortality rates in relation to weekly radiation dose does not preclude the interposition of "biological processes" that influence the carcinogenic and life shortening effects of neutrons (and perhaps other high LET radiations) and most likely the shape of the dose-response curve.

That enhancement occurs with fractionated neutron doses given at low dose rates is of interest as an academic pursuit and in connection with understanding mechanisms in biological factors that come into play in the carcinogenic effects of high LET radiations. The existence of enhancement at doses below 20 rad and the relevance of this phenomenon for the human experience remains to be determined. It is known that neutron dose fractionation results in earlier appearance of lethal pulmonary and Harderian gland tumors, in comparison with the same total single dose, (Figs. 4, 5, 6), and that chromosomal translocations in mouse spermatogonial stem cells are also increased (Fig. 6), but it does not necessarily follow that all tumors will respond in this fashion to neutron dose fractionation. Although Grahn has chosen to fit his chromosome translocation data with

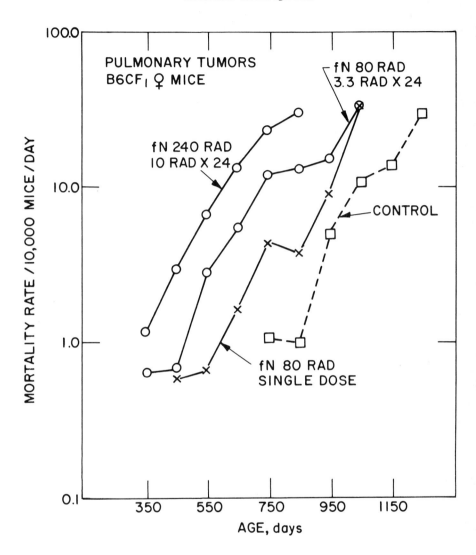

Fig. 4. Age-specific mortality rates from lethal pulmonary tumors in B6CF$_1$ female mice in the Janus program. Reprinted with permission from Ainsworth et al. 1977, reference 58.

linear functions (43), careful inspection of the data for both single and fractionated neutron exposures indicate that curvilinear functions, similar to those described for life shortening, could also be used. At some fission

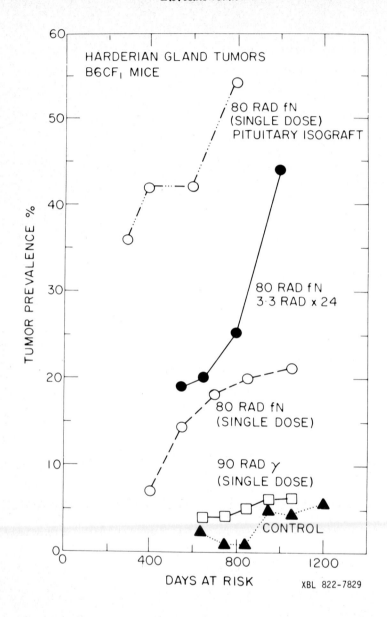

Fig. 5. Prevalence of Harderian gland tumors as a function of the number of days at risk. Mice were irradiated at 100 days of age. The pituitary isografts were carried out at least 4 weeks prior to irradiation. Results from the Janus program from Fry, 1977, reference 59; reprinted with permission.

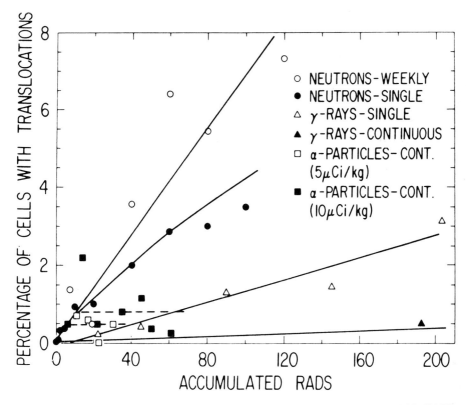

Fig. 6. Reciprocal chromosome translocations induced in the spermatogonia of B6CF$_1$ mice following exposure to JANUS neutrons, ^{60}Co gamma radiations, or alpha particles from ^{239}Pu. Each data point is based on evaluation of 500 to 1000 cells. Although the authors used linear regressions to fit many of the data, it should be noted that the initial slope of the dose-response curves for both single and fractionated neutron doses is quite high and the slope of the response tends to diminish at higher doses, perhaps above 20-40 neutron rad. As with life shortening, and the response of some tumors, the response could be curvilinear, and dose fractionations produces an enhanced response among surviving cells showing translocations. Note also that the response to ^{239}Pu alpha particles is high at the lowest dose rate evaluated, and diminishes dramatically at total accumulated doses above about 20 rad. Reprinted with permission from Grahn et al., 1977, reference 43.

neutron doses, H. H. Vogel Jr. has observed an enhancement in the incidence of mammary tumors in Sprague-Dawley rats when doses were given over 30 days, rather than a single dose (personal communication). Enhancement has also been described for injury to coronary blood vessels in the mouse heart (42). Because vascular tissues are not considered to be characterized by a high rate of cell proliferation, the enhancement phenomenon occurs in both rapidly and slowly dividing mouse tissues. Enhancement of cell killing by high LET radiations may occur, as has been described in the testes by DeRuiter-Bootsma, *et al.* (45) and Goldstein *et al.* (46) but the life shortening, carcinogenic, and chromosomal effects described above characterize the *responses in surviving cells.* Dead cells do not cause cancer, but cell population perturbations resulting from cell killing could influence proliferation rates and the expression of neoplastic transformations in proliferative tissues. Han and associates have also made important observations of neutron dose rate effects on transformation. A 5-7 fold increase in transformed cells occurs when the dose rate is decreased from 15 to less than 1 rad/min (Han, personal communication). Low dose rates/fraction were used in all the Janus mouse experiments, including those on Harderian gland carcinogenesis, so both low dose rate and fractionation could be involved in enhancement of life shortening and carcinogenesis *in vivo.* Elucidation of the mechanism for enhancement must come from colloquy between physicists and biologists because the physical and biological processes may well be involved. Fractionated doses of neutrons may produce cellular and tissue injuries such that recruitment of proliferative cells occurs, the net result being that the population of cells at risk for neoplastic transformations, chromosome aberrations, or expression of other deleterious effects is increased. The extent to which qualitative differences in DNA damage and repair could play some role in cellular and tissue responses after fractionated doses of high LET neutron radiation or gamma radiation is the subject speculation, although it is well known that the RBE for cell division delay is higher than the RBE for cell killing (47). An operational model, if that is the appropriate term, has been proposed by Scott and Ainsworth (48), and deals with the implications of the shape of the dose response curve for life shortening after single doses of neutrons in comparison with the effects of gamma radiation. If indeed a power function is the appropriate curve fit, and the high initial slope is regained between radiation fractions, it follows implicitly that the effects of dose fractionation could be greater than the effects of the same single neutron dose. Although that model contributes little to the understanding of biological mechanisms, implicit within the model is a proposition that a dose-response curve characterized or fitted appropriate by a power function raises the interesting possibility of enhancement as a consequence of dose fractionation or administration of a dose at low dose rates using a continuous exposure design.

9. Tumor Dose-Response Curves

The proposition that different tumor types in mouse (or man) would be expected to respond differently in relation to dose or LET is described best by the results published recently from the Oak Ridge National Laboratory by Dr. Ullrich and associates (39, 40). The effects of dose, dose rate, and radiation quality differ appreciably when thymic lymphomas and pituitary tumors are compared (Figs. 7, 8). It is noteworthy that the curvilinear neutron dose-response relationships observed by Ullrich *et al.* for thymic lymphomas (39) is similar to shape of the chromosomal aberration curve reported by Grahn (43) and the curves for life shortening published by Ainsworth *et al.* (8), Thomson *et al.* (5, 9), and Storer *et al.* (49). Because the experimental design utilized by Ullrich and associates involves a constant dose rate in variable duration of exposure, one can only speculate on the extent to which the enhancement phenomena is influenced by the duration of perturbations produced in cell populations by repeated exposures to fractionated doses of fission neutrons or other high LET radiations. Enhancement of life shortening and thymic lymphoma incidence was seen only at high doses administered over several months (31, 32). The proposition that different cells/tissues at risk to radiation carcinogenesis may differ in response to fractionated doses of high LET radiations is supported by the data of Ullrich *et al.* when the frequency of pituitary

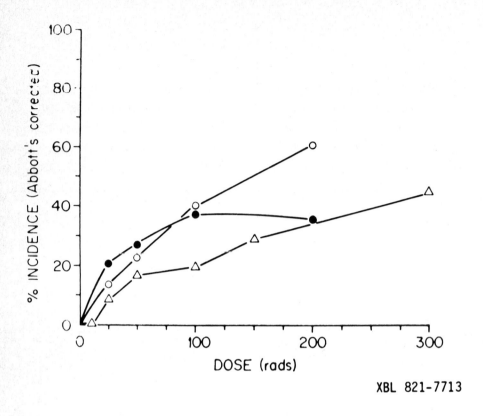

Fig. 7. Percent incidence of thymic leukemia in female RFM mice irradiated at 12 weeks of age. Mice were given single doses of fission-spectrum neutrons from the HPRR reactor (●), chronic neutron exposures at 0.96rad/20hr. day (○), or single doses of ^{60}Cobalt gamma rays (△). Reprinted from Ullrich et al., 1976, reference 39.

tumors is considered (Fig. 8). Even when the duration of exposure was long (1.0 rad/day administered at low dose rates) there was no evidence of pituitary tumor enhancement; to the contrary, the data are consistent with a significant sparing effect at doses of 50 and 20 rad. One could speculate that the cell population kinetics of the tissue at risk, or a particular tissue's responsiveness to radiation damage, in the homeostatic sense, determines

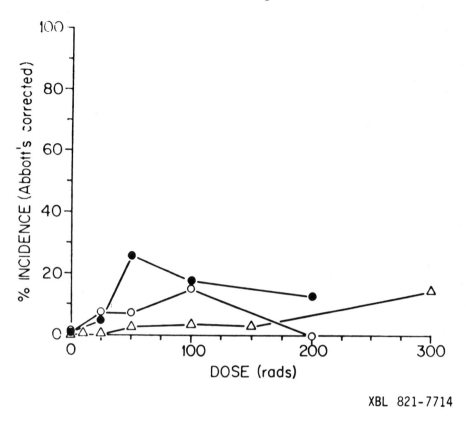

Fig. 8. Adjusted percent incidence of pituitary tumors in female RFM mice irradiated at 12 weeks of age. Mice were given single doses of fission-spectrum neutrons from the HPRR reactor (●), chronic neutron exposures at 0.96rad/20hr. day (○), or single doses of ^{60}Cobalt gamma rays (Δ). Reprinted with permission from Ullrich et al., 1976, reference 39.

the extent to which the size of cell populations at risk may be increased, and the likelihood of enhancement of neoplastic diseases by neutron dose fractionation.

Results on Harderian Gland Carcinogenesis

Tumor model systems were described briefly above, and I would like now to call attention to a very interesting model system, andenocarcinoma of the Harderian gland, which has been explored most extensively by Fry and his colleagues (29, 50). The Harderian gland is a small secretory gland located behind the eye of many rodent species, and radiation-induced Harderian gland tumors had been known for nearly three decades. It is noteworthy that the shape of the dose response curve following exposure to fission neutron radiation, either at Argonne or at Oak Ridge National Laboratory, may be "convexed upward" for the Harderian gland tumor, as is the case for the life shortening response in the mice exposed to neutrons at Argonne. Fry has shown the maximum tumor incidence is reached at a comparatively low dose (40-60 fission neutron rad), and with increasing neutron dose, the total lifetime incidence either increases only slightly or decreases with somewhat higher doses (Fig. 9). Higher energy neutrons are less effective and the maximum incidence occurs at 160 rad. The shape of the gamma radiation curve for this tumor is probably linear at least over a dose range from a few to approximately 270 gamma rad (50). After a single dose of neutrons, the RBE is comparatively high, 12-16 at 20 rad. Other interesting properties of this tumor are that among unirradiated controls the total life time incidence is low, about 3%, and the tumor occurs late in the control life span. Interestingly, over the range of fission neutron or gamma radiation doses studied so far, the peak tumor incidence observed after neutron irradiation (about 17%) is probably higher than the peak incidence observed after gamma radiation. The reason for this is not currently understood but could involve qualitative differences in the type of radiation damage produced. It should be noted parenthetically that, in terms of transformed cells per survivor, Han and Elkind have also found a higher maximum frequency for neutrons than for photons (51). In addition to LET dependence on the shapes of the dose-response curves and the maximum tumor incidents produced, a LET dependence is also noted in terms of the degree of malignancy of this tumor (15). Unirradiated control animals rarely, if ever, show metastasis to the lung or invasion of the

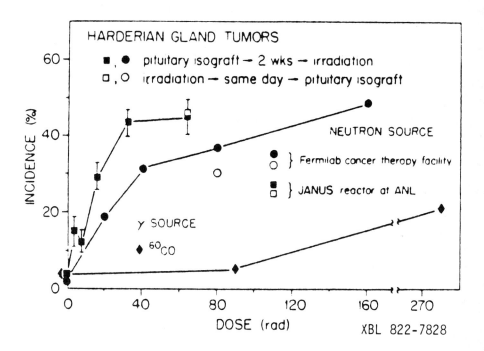

Fig. 9. The incidence of Harderian gland tumors as a function of dose by JANUS reactor fission neutrons (□), (■); Fermi Lab neutron facility neutrons (●), (○), and ^{60}Cobalt gamma radiation (♦) in B6CF$_1$ female mice with pituitary isografts. JANUS is a 200KV water-cooled and moderated reactor; the neutrons have a mean energy of 0.85MeV. The Fermi Facility neutrons are produced by a 65MeV proton beam on a beryllium target and have a mean energy of 25MeV. Reprinted with permission from Fry 1981, reference 50.

cranium. In contrast, the probability of metastasis is increased in irradiated animals, and the frequency of metastasis is different for neutron and gamma irradiated animals. Where the endpoint is the frequency of lethal (metastasizing) Harderian gland tumors over the total number of Harderian gland tumors, the frequency of lethal tumors is weakly dependent, if at all, on gamma radiation dose and ranges from about 8-11% over a single dose range of 90-800 rad. Over the single dose range of 20-240 neutron rad, the frequency of lethal tumors rises from 10% to approximately 30%, and when a total of 240 neutron rad is administered in 24 fractions over 23 weeks, the frequency of lethal tumors rises to 40% (15). If gamma radiation doses are administered at low dose rates over long periods of time, as was described above for the JANUS experiments, the frequency of lethal Harderian gland tumors shows a tendency to decrease. Life-span studies of age-specific prevalence of Harderian gland tumors show that radiation produces a dose-dependent decrease in latent period, relationship being that higher the dose, the shorter the latent period (46).

Another very interesting property of the Harderian gland tumor is the influence of the pituitary gland hormone, prolactin, on expression of this tumor. Fry *et al.* have shown that radiation and prolactin acts synergistically on expression of this tumor (29, 50). Transplantation of two pituitary glands from mice of the same strain to a location beneath spleen capsule results in elevated blood levels of prolactin, because in the spleen, the pituitary is remote from the other anatomical/hormonal influences within the brain that influence regulation of hormone levels. Pituitary transplantation does not influence total life time incidence or latent period of Harderian gland tumors in unirradiated control animals, but the total incidence and latent period changed markedly among irradiated animals. At approximately 800 days at risk, the prevalence is approximately 20% in animals that received a single 80 rad neutron dose, whereas, the prevalence at that time exceeds 50% when animals received a pituitary transplant before irradiation. Fry has demonstrated that the effect of pituitary transplantation, and the accompanying hormone excess, is on tumor expression, rather than alteration of the susceptibility of the gland to neoplastic transformation. Transplantation following irradiation produces the same increased incidence and shortening of the latent period (50). It should be noted also that the Harderian gland tumor also shows enhancement following neutron dose fractionation based on tumor prevalence: at approximately 1000 days at risk, the prevalence was approximately 22% among the animals that received a single 80 rad neutron dose, but at this time the prevalence was approximately 45% among the animals that received 24 fractions of 3.3 neutron rad (50).

The synergistic effect between ionizing radiation and the hormone prolactin is of great interest in itself, but because of the increased rate of tumor expression, we are provided with a model system whereby shapes of dose-response curves can probably be determined accurately over a range of "low doses". Accurate determination of the initial slopes of dose-response curves will yield estimates of RBE for tumor induction. Fry has pointed the shape of the neutron dose-response curve for Harderian gland tumors, with and without pituitary transplantation, differs (50). As is the case for lifespan shortening, and production of chromosome aberrations in mouse spermatogonia, the shapes of the dose-response curves for incidence of Harderian gland tumors appear convexed upwards when no transplants are involved; however, following transplantation, the shape of the dose-response curve appears linear over the initial portion of the curve. Critical comparisons between curve shapes may provide means by which to establish dose-response relationships for "induction or transformation", in comparison with shape of dose-response curves for tumor expression. Interesting comparisons should be possible between shapes of dose-response curves for cell cultures transformed *in vitro*, and shapes of dose-response curves for "transformations that result in Harderian gland tumors". Such studies should contribute materially to improving our understanding of some of the biological factors considered to be important in radiation carcinogenesis.

10. LET Dependence of Harderian Gland Carcinogenesis: Work in Progress

Fry and his associates have embarked on a series of experiments, using the Harderian gland system with pituitary transplants, to determine the LET dependence for tumor induction over a range of low radiation doses. Using this model system, Fry, Alpen, and associates are conducting experiments where mice have been exposed to photons, neutrons of various energies (Fig. 9), or heavy charged particles (from the Bevalac acceleratory at the Lawrence Berkeley Laboratory (52, 53)). A wide range of dose-averaged LETs is represented. As mentioned earlier in this presentation, the question of the appropriate quality factor to use for estimation of risk of radiation carcinogenesis is currently related to the LET of that radiation. RBE-LET relationships for cell transformation *in vitro* or carcinogenesis *in vivo* are not yet fully described over a wide range of LETs. Early work by Hirono using the plant system *Arabidopsis* indicated that peak somatic mutation and tumor induction rates were reached at LET values somewhere between 60 and 200 KeV/μm (54). The RBE for tumor induction at the peak (33) was higher than the peak RBE for induction of somatic mutations (22). Additionally, between a LET of 60 and 200 KeV/μm, the RBE for somatic mutation declined, whereas the RBE for tumor induction remained high. Thus, as you will doubtlessly hear later at this meeting, RBEs for mutagenesis and tumor induction may not be the same, and the extent to which mutagenesis either *in vitro* or *in vivo* can be used to predict tumor induction is a subject for much further discussion. Cox *et. al.* have recently provided qualitatively similar results on mutation induction in comparison with cell killing, for both human and hamster cells *in vitro* (55). Based on results available from several systems, RBE for tumor induction would be expected to diminish after some level of LET, say 200 KeV/μm, is exceeded. Two of the heavy charged-particle beams for which data are available are characterized by dose-averaged LETs of 200 KeV/μm or greater. The LET estimated for the plateau portion of 600 MeV iron ions is on the order of 200 KeV/μm, and the LET estimate for stopping argon particles is of the order of 500 KeV/μm. The surprising results are that exposure to plateau iron ions or stopping argon particles results in a high prevalence of Harderian gland tumors. The carcinogenic effects of high LET iron and argon particles are quite high and this departs from conventional wisdom with respect a decline in RBE at "high" values of LET. Because different cells *in situ* exhibit different sensitivities to different ionizing radiations and different RBEs, there is reason to believe, together with ample data, that RBEs and RBE-LET relationships will differ for different tissues where carcinogenesis is the endpoint.

11. Damage Interactions

The preceding section considered RBE-LET relationships, a matter which is fundamental to human risk assessment for carcinogenesis, or any other endpoint of interest. National and international committees make recommendations as to the most appropriate "quality factor" (Q) to be used for radiations of different LET values based on their careful consideration of all data available, including human data. For example, if the total dose sustained is from low-LET radiation, a Q of 1 is assumed, and some level of risk is inferred based on the total dose. In this case dose is expressed in rem units where rem is defined as dose in rad times the quality factor inferred for that radiation quality. Likewise, the situation would not be terribly complicated if the total dose sustained were from high LET radiation, where a Q of greater than 1 would be used. Where the total dose involves a mixture of high and low radiations, the fractions of the high and low LET doses, respectively, are assigned Q values and rem doses, and the effects are assumed to be additive. The concept of additivity is eminently sensible, but certain recent data provide some impetus for further consideration of this matter. Ngo and his associates have tested the hypothesis of independence of high and low LET radiation damage for the killing of V79 hamster cells cultured *in vitro* (56, 57). As an alternative to simultaneous exposures to mixtures of high and low let radiation, fractionated exposures to high and low LET radiations respectively were given where the time interval between doses has been carefully controlled. Fig. 10 shows that when a dose of high LET neon radiation is followed by a dose of low LET X-rays, the shoulder of the X-ray survival curve is reduced in a time-dependent fashion. Cell-cycle changes, together with other mechanisms by which cellular sensitivity is altered may be involved in this phenomenon, but the clear inference is that for *cell killing*, simultaneous exposure to high and low LET radiation could produce a greater level of cell killing than would be inferred from total independence of radiation effects. The extent to which this non-independence, demonstrated convincingly for cell killing, could obtain for other important biological endpoint, such as mutagenesis or carcinogenesis, remains to be determined.

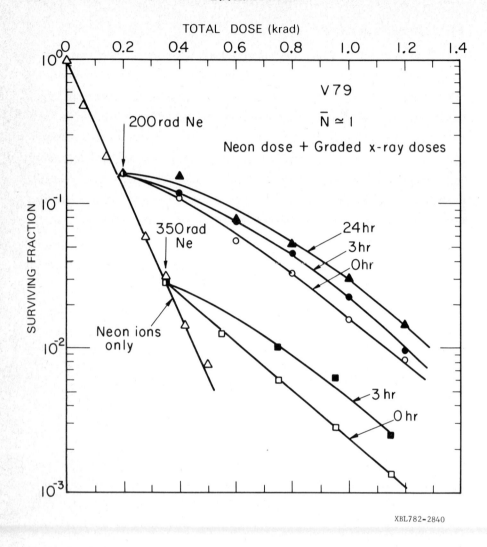

Fig. 10. Survival responses of asynchronized Chinese hamster V79 cells exposed first to 425MeV/amu $^{20}_{10}$Ne ions from the Bevalac, and subsequently to 225KeV X-rays. Reprinted with permission from Ngo et al., 1981, reference 56.

12. Synopsis - The Challenge

This presentation has concentrated on the various physical and biological factors that must be considered in dealing with the problem of radiation carcinogenesis. Items have been stressed in the hope that perspective will be added to the views of this audience when our statistician colleagues, perhaps together with the biologists, attempt to formulate predictive models. Phenomena are described that, I hope, will present a challenge both to the statisticians and radiobiologists in the audience in the context of dealing with mechanisms as well as development of predictive models for radiation carcinogenesis.

Let me now summarize briefly some of the phenomena that I have considered above that I would like the modelers in the audience to consider:

1. Do results from the JANUS experiments inferring linear-quadratic relationships for the expectation of life shortening provide dose-response relationships for life shortening that depart from those expectations? The neutron dose-response curve is "convex upwards", conforms to a slope of approximately 0.6 on a log-log plot, and the gamma dose response curve does not present a strong quadratic component.

2. Fractionation of a fission neutron dose increases the life shortening effect and least certain tumors appear earlier. It is not clear at this time the extent to which this effect is attributable to cell-cycle population alterations that increase the number of cells at risk for carcinogenesis; i.e., a recruitment, or the extent to which the effect is related to promotional effects of repeated radiation damage on expression of carcinogenesis. Estimates of the degree of enhancement are considered conservative, because the alterations in survival time or expression of age-dependent frequencies of tumors are queued from the time the *first* fractionated exposure is given.

3. Fractionation of a gamma radiation dose does not decrease the magnitude of the life shortening effect as much as might be expected, and at dose levels of 417 or 206 rad, the sparing of dose fractionation over 20% of life span was not demonstrated.

4. Those elements of the Sacher model that had been interpreted from the linear shape of the dose-response curve to indicate the absence of dose-rate effects for gamma radiation have not been confirmed. Results from the JANUS experiments have indicated that over that range of doses, administering a given weekly dose in fractions rather than at low dose rates over longer periods of time produce greater life shortening than is produced by administering the gamma dose at lower dose rates. This demonstrates convincingly the operation of certain repair processes at low gamma dose rate, over at least some range of radiation doses.

5. Different tumors exhibit different dose-response relationships after single or protracted radiation doses, and these tissue-dependent differences may involve both susceptibility to and expression of neoplastic transformations.

6. The duration of life span over which the radiation dose is given influences appreciably the degree of life shortening and the carcinogenic effect. The susceptible period occurs during the first 50% of the animal's control life span, and the age-dependent susceptibility to radiation-induced life shortening in carcinogenesis may well be dependent upon radiation quality.

7. LET-RBE relationships for carcinogenesis differ in certain important respects from LET-RBE relationships for radiation-induced cell killing because ionizations produced by plateau iron and stopping argon particles where the LET is of the order of 200-600 KeV/m are quite effective in producing Harderian gland tumors.

8. Damage interactions occur for cell killing in such a fashion that the effects of high and low LET doses are not totally independent. Should this happen for carcinogenic or mutagenic endpoints, at low total levels of dose, estimates of risk must be reassessed.

In model development, our statistician colleagues must consider the physics of dose deposition, DNA damage/repair/cell proliferation/cell killing, and matters of dose-rate effects, LET, and the fraction of he life span over which dose is given. Tumor latency and tumor expression represent important and complex biological factors in the influence of various promoters such as cell turnover, viruses, or other substances in the environment which also must be considered. Other important biological factors are the species and the matter of appreciation of tissue differences in susceptibility to and expression of carcinogenic effects of ionizing radiations. Implicit within the development of any models that will contribute to our understanding of mechanisms and provide means by which cancer risk may be estimated is careful consideration of dose-response relationships for cancer induction and expression. To paraphrase a statement Prof. Neyman has made in another context, let me say that, as an intellectual pursuit, the scientific question of radiation carcinogenesis is very complicated, but not uninteresting.

Effort devoted to preparation of this manuscript was supported by the U.S. Department of Energy and NASA.

13. References

1. National Academy of Sciences. *Biological Effects of Ionizing Radiation.* (The "BEIR Committee" Report, BEIR III), 1980.

2. Fry, R.J.M. Extrapolation from animal systems to man: A review of the problems and possibilities. *Proc. of the Public Meeting March 10-11, 1980 to Address a Proposed Federal Radiation Research Agenda,* Vol 1, *Issue Papers,* pp. 111-136, 1980.

3. Burns, F.J. Somatic effects-cancer. *Proc. of the Public Meeting March 10-11, 1980 to Address a Proposed Federal Radiation Research Agenda.* Vol 2, *Science Projection Papers,* pp. 273-298, 1980.

4. Sacher, G.A. Dose, Dose Rate Radiation Quality and Host Factors for Radiation-Induced Life Shortening. In: *Aging, Carcinogenesis and Radiation Biology: The Role of Nucleic Acid Addition Reactions,* edited by K. C. Smith, New York, Plenum Press, pp. 493-517, 1976.

5. Thomson, J.F., F.S. Williamson, D. Grahn and E.J. Ainsworth. Life shortening in mice exposed to fission neutrons and gamma rays. 1. Single and short-term fractionated exposures. *Radiat. Res.*, Vol 86: 559-572, 1981.

6. National Council on Radiation Protection and Measurements. *Influence of Dose and its Distribution in Time on Dose-Effect Relationships for Low-LET Radiation*, NCRP Report No. 64 (1980).

7. Neary, G.J., R.J. Munson and R.H. Mole. *Chronic Radiation Hazards*, Pergamon, New York, 1957.

8. Ainsworth, E.J., R.J.M. Fry, D. Grahn, F.S. Williamson, P.C. Brennan, S.P. Stearner, A.V. Carrano and J.H. Rust. Late Effects of Neutron or Gamma Irradiation on Mice. In: *Biological Effects of Neutron Irradiation*, International Atomic Energy Agency, Vienna, Austria, pp. 359-379, 1974.

9. Thomson, J.F., F.S. Williamson, D. Grahn and E.J. Ainsworth. Life shortening in mice exposed to fission neutrons and gamma rays. II. Duration-of-Life and long-term fractionated exposures, *Radiat. Res.*, Vol 86: 573-579, 1981.

10. Blakely, E.A., F.Q.H. Ngo, S.B. Curtis and C.A. Tobias. Heavy Ion Radiation Biology: Cellular Studies. *Advances in Radiation Biology*, (in press) 1982.

11. Leith, J.T., E.J. Ainsworth and E.L. Alpen. Radiation Biology of Heavy Ions: Effects on Normal Tissues. *Advances in Radiation Biology*, (in press) 1982.

12. Blakely, E.A., C.A. Tobias, F.Q.H. Ngo and S.B. Curtis. Physical and Cellular Radiobiological Properties of Heavy Ions in Relation to Cancer Therapy Applications. In: *Biological and Medical Research with Accelerated Heavy Ions at the Bevalac,* 1977-1980. Lawrence Berkeley Laboratory (LBL) Report No. 11220, edited by M.C Pirruccello and C.A. Tobias, pp. 73-86, November, 1980.

13. Madhvanath, U., M.R. Raju and L.S. Kelly. Survival of human lymphocytes after exposure to densely ionizing radiations. *ERDA Symposium Series 37,* pp. 125-139, 1976.

14. Grahn, D. and G.A. Sacher. Fractionation and Protraction Factors and the Late Effects of Radiation in Small Mammals. In: *Dose Rate in Mammalian Radiation Biology,* edited by D. G. Brown, R. G. Cragle and T. R. Noonan, Proc. Symp. USAEC Agricultural Research Lab., Oak Ridge, Tennessee, USAEC Conf. 680410, 1968.

15. Fry, R.J.M. and E.J. Ainsworth. Radiation injury: Some aspects of the oncogenic effects, *Fed. Proc.,* Vol 36: 1703-1707, 1977.

16. Upton, A.C., F.F. Wolff, J. Furth and A.W. Kimball. A comparison of the induction of myeloid and lymphoid leukemias in X-irradiated RF mice, *Cancer Res.,* Vol 18: 842-848, 1958.

17. Storer, J.B. Radiation Carcinogenesis. In: *Cancer,* edited by F.F. Becker, Vol 1, Plenum Press, New York, pp. 453-483, 1975.

18. Walburg, H.E. Jr. and G.E. Cosgrove. Life shortening and cause of death in irradiated germ free mice, *Proc. First European Symposium on Late Effects of Radiation,* edited by P. Metalli, pp. 51-67, 1970.

19. Ames, B., W.E. Durston, E. Yamasaki and F.D. Lee. Carcinogens are mutagens: A simple test for combining liver homogenates for activation and bacteria for detection, *Proc. Natl. Acad. Sci. USA*, Vol 70: 2281-2285, 1973.

20. Weisburger, J.H. and G.M. Williams. Carcinogen testing. Current problems and new approaches, *Science*, Vol 214: 401-407, 1981.

21. Hall, E.J. What is the current knowledge about the effects of differences in schedules of delivery of a given dose of ionizing radiation (dose rate, fractionation) and "quality" of radiation (LET) on biological systems and how can this information be used to predict the effects of low doses in man? *Proc. of the Public Meeting March 10-11, 1980 To Address a Proposed Federal Radiation Research Agenda*, Vol 1, Issue paper No. 4, pp. 137-170.

22. Elkind, M.M. What is our current knowledge from animal and cellular systems about the combined effects of ionizing radiation and exposure to other agents (chemicals, pharmacological, physical, viral etc.) and is this knowledge adequate to predict human responses? *Proc. of the Public Meeting March 10-11, 1980, To Address a Proposed Federal Radiation Research Agenda*, Vol 1, Issue paper No. 5, pp. 171-191.

23. Han, A. and M.M. Elkind. Transformation of mouse C3H10T½ cells by single and fractionated doses of X-rays and fission spectrum neutrons, *Cancer Res.*, Vol 39: 123-130, 1979.

24. Miller, R.C., E.J. Hall and H.H. Rossi. Oncogenic transformation of mammalian cells *in vitro* with split-doses of X-rays, *Proc. Natl. Acad. Sci. USA*, Vol 76: 5755-5758, 1979.

25. Borek, C., D.L. Guernsey and A. Ong. Thyroid hormone regulation of radiation and chemically induced neoplastic transformation *in vitro*. *Abstracts of papers for the 29th annual meeting of the Radiation Research Society*, Minneapolis, Minn., May 31 - June 4, 1981, abstract Hc-10, pp. 124.

26. Hoel, D.G. and H.E. Walburg, Jr. Statistical analysis of survival experiments, *J. Natl. Cancer Inst.*, Vol 49: 361-372, 1972.

27. Burns, F.J., R.E. Albert and R.D. Heimbach. The RBE for skin tumors and hair follicle damage in the rat following irradiation with alpha-particles and electrons, *Radiat. Res.*, Vol 36: 225-241, 1968.

28. Shellabarger, C.J., D. Chmelevsky and A.M. Kellerer. Induction of mammary neoplasms in the Sprague-Dawley rat by 430-KeV neutrons and X-rays, *J. Natl. Cancer Inst.*, Vol 64: 821-833, 1980.

29. Fry, R.J.M., A.G. Garcia, K.W. Allen, A. Sallese, T.N. Tahmisian, L.S. Lombard and E.J. Ainsworth. The Effect of Pituitary Isografts on Radiation Carcinogenesis in the Mammary and Harderian Glands of Mice. In: *Biological Effects of Low-Level Radiation Pertinent to Protection of Man and His Environment*, Vienna, IAEA, Vol 1, pp. 213-227, 1976.

30. Major, I.R. and R.H. Mole. Myeloid leukemia in X-ray irradiated CBA mice, *Nature*, Vol 272: 455-456, 1978.

31. Ullrich R.L. and J. B. Storer. Influence of Dose, Dose Rate and Radiation Quality on Radiation Carcinogenesis and Life Shortening in RFM and BALB/c mice. In: *Late Biological Effects of Ionizing Radiation*, Vol II, IAEA, Vienna, pp. 95-102, 1978.

32. Ullrich, R.L. and J.B. Storer. Influence of gamma irradiation on the development of neoplastic disease in mice. II. Solid tumors, *Radiat. Res.*, Vol 80: 317-330, 1979.

33. Upton, A.C., J.W. Conklin and R.A. Popp. Influence of age at irradiation on susceptibility to radiation-induced life-shortening in RF mice, radiation and aging, *Proc. of a Colloquium held in Semmering, Austria, June 23-24, 1966*, edited by P.J. Lindop and G.A. Sacher, Taylor and Francis Ltd., London, p. 337, 1966.

34. Jones, D.C.L. and D.J. Kimeldorf. Effect of age at irradiation on life span in the male rat, *Radiat. Res.*, Vol 22: 106-114, 1964.

35. Grahn, D. Biological Effects of Protracted Low Dose Radiation Exposure of Man and Animals. In: *Late Effects of Radiation*, edited by R.J.M. Fry, D. Grahn, M.L. Griem and J.H. Rust, London, Taylor & Francis, pp. 101-136, 1970.

36. Sacher, G.A. and D. Grahn. Survival of mice under duration-of-life exposure to gamma rays. I. The dosage-survival relation and the lethality function, *J. Natl. Cancer Inst.*, Vol 32: 277-321, 1964.

37. Upton, A.C., M.L. Randolph and J.W. Conklin. Late effects of fast neutrons and gamma rays in mice as influenced by the dose rate of irradiation: Life shortening, *Radiat. Res.*, Vol 32: 493-509, 1967.

38. Upton, A.C., M.L. Randolph and J.W. Conklin. Late effects of fast neutrons and gamma rays in mice as influenced by the dose rate of irradiation: Induction of neoplasia, *Radiat. Res.*, Vol 47: 467-491, 1970.

39. Ullrich, R.L., M.C. Jernigan, G.E. Cosgrove, L. C. Satterfield, N.D. Bowles and J. B. Storer. The influence of dose and dose rate on the incidence of neoplastic disease in RFM mice after neutron irradiation, *Radiat. Res.* Vol 68: 115-131, 1976.

40. Ullrich, R.L. and J.B. Storer. Influence of dose, dose rate and radiation quality on radiation carcinogenesis and life shortening in RFM and BALB/c mice. *Proc. International Symposium on Biological Implications of Radionuclides Released from Nuclear Industries, 26-30 March, 1979*, Vol II, pp. 95-113, International Atomic Energy Agency, Vienna.

41. Kellerer, A.M. and H.H. Rossi. Biophysical aspects of radiation carcinogenesis. In: *Cancer: A Comprehensive Treatise. I. Etiology: Chemical and Physical Carcinogenesis*, edited by F.F. Becker, New York Plenum Press, pp. 405-439, 1975

42. Neary, G.J., E.V. Hulse and R.H. Mole. The relative biological effectiveness of fast neutrons and gamma-rays for life-shortening in chronically irradiated CBA mice, *Inter. J. Radiation Biology*, Vol 4: 239-248, 1962.

43. Grahn, D., B.H. Frystak, C.H. Lee, J.J. Russell and A. Lindenbaum. Dominant lethal mutations and chromosome aberrations induced in male mice by incorporated ^{239}Pu and by external fission neutron and gamma irradiation, *Proc. International Symposium on Biological Implications of Radionuclides Released from Nuclear Industries, March 26-30, 1979*, International Atomic Energy Agency, Vienna, Vol 1, pp. 163-184, 1979.

44. Yang, V.V., S.P. Stearner and E.J. Ainsworth. Late ultrastructural changes in the mouse coronary arteries and aorta after fission neutron or ^{60}Co gamma irradiation, *Radiat. Res.*, Vol 74: 436-456, 1978.

45. De Ruiter-Bootsma, A.L., M.F. Kramer, D.G. de Rooij and J.A.G. Davids. Survival of spermatogonial stem cells in the mouse after split-dose irradiation with fission neutrons of 1-MeV mean energy: Effect of the fractionation interval, *Radiat. Res.*, Vol 79: 289-297, 1979.

46. Goldstein, L.S., T.L. Phillips and G.Y. Ross. Biological effects of accelerated heavy ions. II. Fractionated irradiations of intestinal crypt cells, *Radiat. Res.*, Vol 86: 542-558, 1981.

47. Schneier, D.O. and G.F. Whitmore. Comparative effects of neutrons and X-rays on mammalian cells, *Radiat. Res.*, Vol 18: 286-306, 1963.

48. Scott, R.B. and E.J. Ainsworth. State-vector model for life shortening in mice after brief exposures to low doses of ionizing radiation, *Mathematical Biosciences*, Vol 49: 185-205, 1980.

49. Storer, J.B., L.J. Serrano, E.B. Darden, Jr., M.C. Jernigan and R.L. Ullrich. Life shortening in RFM and BALB/c mice as a function radiation quality, dose, and dose rate, *Radiat. Res.*, Vol 78: 122-161, 1979.

50. Fry, R.J.M. Experimental radiation carcinogenesis: What have we learned? *Radiat. Res.*, Vol 87: 224-239, 1981.

51. Han, A. and M.M. Elkind. The effect of radiation quality and repair processes on the incidence of neoplastic transformation *in vitro*. In: *Radiation Research, Proceedings of the Sixth International Congress of Radiation Research, Tokyo, May 13-19, 1979*, edited by S. Okada, M. Imamura, T. Terasima and H. Yamaguchi, Japanese Association for Radiation Research, Tokyo, 1979.

52. Alpen, E.L., R.J.M. Fry, P. Powers-Risius and E.J. Ainsworth. Carcinogenesis with heavy ion radiation in the Harderian gland of mice. In: *Biological and medical Research with Accelerated Heavy Ions at the Bevalac, 1977-1980*, Lawrence Berkeley Laboratory (LBL), Report No. 11220, edited by M.C. Pirruccello and C.A. Tobias, pp. 255-260, November, 1980.

53. Powers-Risius, P., E.L. Alpen, R.J.M. Fry and E.J. Ainsworth. Harderian gland carcinogenesis by heavy ions. *Abstracts of papers for the 29th annual meeting of the Radiation Research Society*, Minneapolis, Minn., May 31 - June 4, 1981. pp. 79, abstract Fc-10.

54. Hirono, Y., H.H. Smith, J.T. Lyman, K.H. Thompson, and J.W. Baum. Relative biological effect of heavy ions in producing mutations, tumors and growth inhibition in the crucifer plant *Arabidopsis, Radiat. Res.*, Vol 44: 204-223, 1970.

55. Cox, T., J. Thacker, D.T. Goodhead and R.J. Munson. Mutation and inactivation of mammalian cells by various ionizing radiations, *Nature* (London), Vol 267: 425-427, 1977.

56. Ngo, F.Q.H., A. Han and M.M. Elkind. On the repair of sublethal damage in V79 Chinese hamster cells resulting from irradiation with neutrons combined with X-rays. *Inter. J. Radiation Biology*, Vol 32: 507-511, 1977.

57. Ngo, F.Q.H., E.A. Blakely and C.A. Tobias. Sequential exposures of mammalian cells to low and high LET radiations. I. Lethal effects following X-ray and neon-ion irradiation, *Radiat. Res.*, Vol 87: 59-78, 1981.

58. Ainsworth, E.J., R.J.M. Fry, F.S. Williamson, P.C. Brennan, S.P. Stearner, V.V. Yang, D.A. Crouse, J.H. Rust and T.B. Bovak. Dose-effect relationships for life-shortening, tumorigenesis and systemic injuries in mice irradiated with fission neutron or ^{60}Co gamma radiation, *Proc. IVth International Congress*, International Radiation Protection Association, Vol 4, pp. 1143-1151, 1977.

59. Fry, R.J.M. Radiation carcinogenesis. Particles and radiation therapy, Second International Conference, *International J. Radiat. Oncol. Biol. Phys.*, Vol 3: 219-226, 1977.

A Hypothetical Stochastic Mechanism of Radiation Effects in Single Cells: Some Further Thoughts and Results

Prem S. Puri[*]

Dept. of Statistics, Purdue University
West Lafayette, Indiana 47907

1. Introduction.

The purpose of the present paper is to briefly describe a stochastic model for radiation effects in single cells recently studied by J. Neyman and the author (see [9], [10]), discuss some results based on this model and then raise several questions which need further attention. At the outset it is appropriate to mention that originally we were inspired by the experimental work on animals such as mice, particularly that due to Upton, et al ([16],[17]). However reading through the literature we soon realized the complexity of the various mechanisms that together appear to play role in bringing about variety of responses from animals as a result of their exposure to radiation. While our ultimate goal is to develop appropriate stochastic models of phenomena arising in irradiated experimental animals, our present concern however is limited to irradiation effects on cells of some homogeneous tissue.

The literature on this subject is quite rich. The closest ancestor to our stochastic model appears in the work of Payne and Garret ([11],[12]). Our model differs from this and others in two basic details described below.

The source of irradiation emits particles, which we label "primary". When a single particle crosses a living cell, it generates a cluster of particles

---
[*]These investigations were supported in part by the U. S. National Science Foundation Grant No. MCS-8102733.

that we label "secondary". The sizes of clusters vary with the kind of irradiation. Clusters generated by low linear energy transfer (LET) radiation primaries (such as those of X-rays, gamma rays, etc.) contain few secondaries, while those generated by high LET primaries (such as those of α-particles and neutrons) contain many secondaries. It is visualized that the irradiation damage to cells is mainly due to the secondary particles that "hit" the sensitive parts of living cells. The second detail of the chance mechanism is concerned with what may be called the time scales of radiation damage and of subsequent repair. The generation of a cluster of secondary particles and the possible hits occur so rapidly that for all practical purposes, they may be considered as occurring instantly. On the other hand, the subsequent changes in the damaged cells, such as repair, etc., appear to require measurable amounts of time.

We begin in the next section with the basic assumptions that underlie our stochastic model. In section 3, we qualitatively compare some of the implications of our model with the empirical findings available in literature. Section 4 deals with the case of UV-radiation, where the question of whether or not a primary particle of UV-radiation generates any secondary is touched upon. Finally we close with section 5, where we raise several questions of interest that are either under study or need further attention.

2. Stochastic Model of Radiation Effects on Single Cells.

We consider a hypothetical experiment in which a live cell is subjected to a particular kind of irradiation. The irradiation is assumed to be administered over T units of time at a constant dose-rate, denoted by ρ. The time T is such that by the end of this time a preassigned total dose of irradiation, measured in rads and denoted by D, is given so that $D = \rho T$. The specific assumptions of our stochastic model are as follows.

(A_1) Primary radiation particles arrive at the cell according to a Poisson process with rate $\lambda(t)$ per unit of time and per unit volume, where $\lambda(t) = \lambda > 0$, for $0 \leqslant t \leqslant T$ and $\lambda(t) = 0$, for $t > T$.

(A_2) Each primary generates a cluster of secondary particles, the number of which, denoted by ν, is a random variable. It is assumed that the numbers ν of secondaries generated by several primaries are mutually independent with a common distribution having a finite mean ν_1.

(A_3) The secondary particles of a cluster are assumed to travel independently of each other and independently from all other variables of the system.

(A_4) Within each live cell we visualize two disjoint "targets", the biological identity of which we do not attempt to specify. Possibly they can be some particular points within a chromosome, etc. These targets are denoted by R and K, connoting "repairable" and "killing". Both targets are located in a region within the cell, denoted by A, connoting region of "accessibility". We postulate that the passage of a primary radiation particle outside the region A has no effect on the cell considered. On the other hand, if a primary particle crosses A, then each of the ν generated secondaries has the same probabilities π_1 and π_2 of hitting the targets R or K, respectively. It will be convenient to use the same letter A to designate the volume of the region of accessibility A.

(A_5) The generation of a cluster of secondaries by a single primary particle and the subsequent possible hits on R and K occur instantaneously.

The above assumptions (A_1)-(A_5) concern the physical aspects of our stochastic model. We now turn to its biological aspects.

(A_6) If the target R is hit by a secondary particle, the cell experiences a "repairable" damage. We abstain from specifying the mechanism of repair, which may involve enzymes, etc. Under the Markovian assumption, given that a cell at time t is alive and has a nonnegative number k of unrepaired hits of target R, we assume that

(i) the conditional probability of a single damage being repaired in (t,t+h) is $\alpha k h + o(h)$;

(ii) the conditional probability of a repairable damage becoming permanent (nonlethal) in (t,t+h) is $\beta k h + o(h)$;

(iii) the conditional probability of a repairable damage becoming (lethal) in (t,t+h) is $\gamma k h + o(h)$;

(iv) the conditional probability of the cell dying in (t,t+h) due to causes not directly connected with radiation is $\delta h + o(h)$; and

(v) the conditional probability of more than one of the above events happening in (t,t+h) is $o(h)$.

Here α, β, γ, and δ designate nonnegative possibly time dependent functions of which δ may also depend on the dose rate ρ. In (ii) the biological nature of the permanent damage is not specified, but judging from relevant literature it will frequently consist in the cell's becoming the first of an initiated development of some cancer. For this reason, in [9] and [10], it was felt convenient to speak of this damage as "cancerous". However, recently we have learnt that in radiation research literature cells with such damages are more commonly referred to as "transformed" cells. This appears more appropriate since not all transformed cells are in general cancerous. Thus from here-on we shall also use this same terminology when referring to such cells.

(A_7) Regarding the target K, we assume that a single hit causes the death (or inactivation) of the cell. Similarly a single lethal damage of type (iii) above also causes its inactivation. Thus the cell could die either due to a hit on the target K, or due to the risk γ in (iii) or due to the risk δ in (iv). Finally, a live cell is considered transformed as soon as a permanent damage results due to the risk β in (ii).

In [10], we have considered the more general case, where the rates λ, α, β, γ and δ may be time dependent. However for the present, we shall consider only the case where they are constant, while keeping the risk δ of death due to other causes dependent on the dose rate ρ at which the irradiation is applied.

Again it was felt appropriate to assume that the mean number ν_1 of secondary particles produced by a single primary particle is directly proportional to the initial energy of the particle. This suggests that the dose rate ρ (radiation energy absorbed per unit time) should approximately be directly proportional to the product $\lambda \nu_1 A$, where λ is the mean number of primary particles arriving per unit time and per unit volume. Thus we may set

$$\lambda \nu_1 A = \theta \rho, \tag{1}$$

where θ is a positive constant, which typically may depend on the energy, mass of the particles, type of radiation involved, etc.

In the next section we present certain formulas derived in [10] under the assumptions (A_1)-(A_7), that are relevant to certain empirical findings against which the implications of these formulas are qualitatively compared. The reader may refer to [10] for their detailed derivation.

3.1. Proportion of Surviving Cells.

Figure 1 (taken from Barendsen [1]) exhibits the behavior of the logarithm of the proportion of the cells surviving immediately following the exposure of a total radiation dose D (measured in rads) when plotted against this dose. In general, it is a decreasing function of D, but its behavior varies with the type of radiation. For instance, for high LET radiation such as neutrons or α-particles, this plot is almost like a straight line. On the other hand, for the low LET radiation this plot is nonlinear and shows a degree of concavity, commonly referred to as the "shouldering effect". The theoretical analog of the proportion of surviving cells at time t corresponds to the probability of a cell to be alive at time t. The logarithm of this probability, subject to the assumptions of our model and the relation (1), is given by

$$\ln P(\text{cell is alive at } t) = \tag{2}$$

$$-t\delta(\rho) - \frac{\theta \rho}{\nu_1} \int_{\max(0, t-D/\rho)}^{t} \{1 - g(K(\tau))\} d\tau,$$

where the function $g(\cdot)$ is the probability generating function (p.g.f) of the

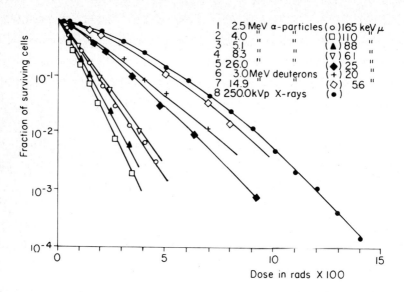

Figure 1. Dose-survival curves of cultured $T-1_g$ cells in equilibrium with air, irradiated with different mono-energetic heavy charged particles in conditions where narrow distributions of dose in LET are obtained. (Taken from Barendsen [1].)

random variable ν, the number of secondaries generated by a primary particle and

$$K(\tau) = 1 - \pi_2 - \frac{\pi_1 \gamma}{\alpha+\beta+\gamma} (1-\exp[-(\alpha+\beta+\gamma)\tau]). \qquad (3)$$

In order to match (2) with the curves in figure 1, we set $t = T = D/\rho$, the exposure time for the total radiation dose D, and obtain from (2)

$\ln P(\text{cell is alive at } T) =$

$$-\frac{\delta(\rho)D}{\rho} - \frac{\theta\rho}{\nu_1} \int_0^{D/\rho} \{1-g(K(\tau))\} d\tau. \qquad (4)$$

Again to study the behavior of (4) as a function of D, we note that the derivative $\partial \ln P/\partial D$ is always negative, so that $\ln P$ is a decreasing function of D. Here P designates the probability P(cell is alive at T) as given in (4). Also as long as $\pi_1\gamma$ is positive, $\partial^2\ln P/\partial D^2$ is negative so that $\ln P$ is strictly a concave function. Consequently its plot may often show some shouldering effect consistent with some of the empirical plots of Figure 1 that correspond to low LET radiation. This effect however is negligible for high LET radiation such as neutrons, where a primary particle whenever it generates any positive number of secondaries, it does so typically in thousands. This being the case, for the high LET radiation, we may take approximately

$$g(s) \approx g(0), \qquad (5)$$

for s not close to one. Since in our case $K(t) \leq 1 - \pi_2$, for all $t \geq 0$, with $\pi_2 > 0$, the approximation (5) used for $g(K(\tau))$ in (4) may not be unreasonable. Thus we have approximately

$$\ln P(\text{cell is alive at } T) \approx -\frac{\delta(\rho)D}{\rho} - \frac{\theta D}{\nu_1}[1-g(0)]. \qquad (6)$$

This being linear in D, explains the absence of shouldering effect for the case of high LET radiation, as observed empirically (see Figure 1).

Again the behavior of the empirical dose-survival curves is known to vary also with the dose rate ρ (see for instance, Bedford and Hall [2] and Hall and Bedford [5]). In [10], it was shown that with an appropriate choice of the function $\delta(\rho)$ the expression (4), treated as a function of ρ, remains qualitatively consistent with the corresponding behavior of empirical curves. The reader may refer to [10] for the relevant details.

3.2. Proportion of Cells Ever Getting Transformed.

To begin with we mention one of the empirical findings in animal experimentation due to Upton, et al. [16] (see Totter [15]), which stimulated our work. This refers to the so called "dose-rate effect" of gamma radiation on the induction of a particular leukemia in mice. It is observed that for the same total dose D given at a high dose rate a substantially higher percentage of irradiated mice acquired leukemia than those given at a low dose rate. Similar results were found by these authors for other cancers. In particular, it is observed in the case of high dose rate, that the incidence of leukemia is not a monotone function of the total dose D. It first increases with increasing dose D, reaches a maximum and then decreases. Since our model refers to cells, later we also found some published work on cells, exhibiting a similar behavior in terms of the incidence of cell transformation as a result of radiation exposure (see for instance, Sparrow et al. [13], Nauman, et al. [8], and Han, Hill and Elkind [7]) (Also see Figure 2).

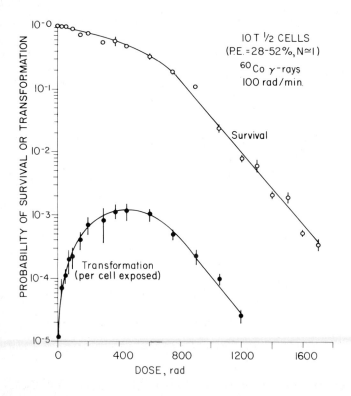

Figure 2. Survival and neoplastic transformation of C3H/10T½ cells by ^{60}Co γ-rays delivered at 100 rads/min. Transformation is expressed per exposed cell. (Taken from Han, Hill and Elkind [7] with the kind permission of the authors and Cancer Research, Inc.)

For the theoretical counterpart of these empirical findings, formulas giving the probability that an irradiated cell ever becomes transformed, were derived in [10] based on our stochastic model. These are reproduced below from [10].

For the case when $\delta(\rho) > 0$, we have

$P(\text{cell ever gets transformed})$

$$= \frac{\beta}{\beta+\gamma} \left\{ 1 - \{\delta(\rho) + \frac{\theta\rho}{\nu_1}[1-g(1-\pi_2)]\} \right. \tag{7}$$

$$\cdot \int_0^{D/\rho} \exp\left[-\delta(\rho)t - \frac{\theta\rho}{\nu_1}\int_0^t \{1-g[R(\tau)]\}\,d\tau\right] dt$$

$$\left. -\delta(\rho) \int_{D/\rho}^{\infty} \exp\left[-\delta(\rho)t - \frac{\theta\rho}{\nu_1}\int_{t-D/\rho}^t \{1-g[R(\tau)]\}\,d\tau\right] dt \right\}.$$

However when $\delta(\rho) = 0$, we have

$P(\text{cell ever gets transformed})$

$$= \frac{\beta}{\beta+\gamma} \left\{ 1 - \frac{\theta\rho}{\nu_1}\{1-g[1-\pi_2]\} \right.$$

$$\cdot \int_0^{D/\rho} \exp\left[-\frac{\theta\rho}{\nu_1}\int_0^t \{1-g[R(\tau)]\}\,d\tau\right] dt \tag{8}$$

$$\left. - \exp\left[-\frac{\theta D}{\nu_1}\{1-g[R(\infty)]\}\right] \right\},$$

where

$$R(\tau) = 1 - \pi_2 - \frac{\pi_1(\beta+\gamma)}{\alpha+\beta+\gamma}\{1-\exp[-(\alpha+\beta+\gamma)t]\} \tag{9}$$

and

$$R(\infty) = 1 - \pi_2 - \frac{\pi_1(\beta+\gamma)}{\alpha+\beta+\gamma}. \tag{10}$$

The study of the expressions (7) and (8) treated as a function of D, leads to the following proposition proved in [10].

PROPOSITION. *Let the rates α, β, γ and $\delta(\rho)$ be all independent of time. Then, under the assumptions $(A_1)-(A_7)$, P(cell ever gets transformed) treated as a function of D has exactly one maximum if and only if*

$$\delta(\rho) \int_0^\infty \exp\left[-\delta(\rho)t - \frac{\theta\rho}{\nu_1}\int_0^{D/\rho}\{g[R(u)] - g[R(u+t)]\}\, du\right] \quad (11)$$

$$\cdot \{1 - g[R(t)]\}\, dt \;<\; 1 - g[1-\pi_2],$$

whenever $\delta(\rho) > 0$, and

$$\exp\left[-\frac{\theta\rho}{\nu_1}\int_0^\infty \{g[R(u)] - g[R(\infty)]\}\, du\right]\{1 - g[R(\infty)]\} \quad (12)$$

$$< \; 1 - g[1-\pi_2],$$

whenever $\delta(\rho) = 0$. Otherwise P(cell ever gets transformed) is an increasing function of D.

As indicated in the above proposition, under appropriate conditions on the parameters exhibited by (11) and (12), our model is consistent with the empirical findings of Upton, et al. [16] and also with those in Figure 2. An interesting fact emerging out of the above proposition is that in our model, in order to have a point of maximum in these curves, it is necessary although not sufficient that π_2 be positive. Evidently it is the competition between the two risks that brings about the point of maximum, one risk being that of the death of the cell through π_2 and the other being the risk of transformation of the cell with rate β. After all, the cells having died due to the risk π_2 are no longer available for becoming transformed, a fact specially significant for high dose levels.

Before closing this section, we remark that in order that our model be consistent with the behavior of the observed dose-response curves for cell transformations for varying dose-rate ρ, it is essential, that $\delta(\rho)$ be positive and have an appropriate dependence on ρ. We refer the reader to [10] for these and other details.

4. The Case of UV-radiation.

The possibility that in the case of UV-radiation a primary particle may itself act as a secondary without really generating any secondaries, was mentioned earlier in [9] and [10]. This of course is equivalent to taking $g(s) = s$ in our case. Perhaps this hypothesis may not be strictly correct. However, in this context, it is worth pointing out that in our model, we have refrained in spelling out the exact physical nature of the entities we labeled as "secondary" particles. May they be ions or free radicals or combinations thereof. Thus whether or not effectively $g(s) = s$ holds in the case of UV-radiation needs further examination based on real data. With suitable data available appropriate statistical tests can be devised to test this hypothesis. For instance, to begin with, we may consider taking

$$g(s) = \frac{\exp[-\xi(1-s)] - \exp[-\xi]}{1 - \exp[-\xi]}, \xi \geq 0, |s| \leq 1. \tag{13}$$

In this case testing the above hypothesis would mean testing the hypothesis that $\xi = 0$, against the alternative that $\xi > 0$. Again the kind of data we anticipate are the following.

At time $t = 0$, a number N of live cells are subjected to a particular kind of radiation administered over time T at a known dose rate ρ, with total preassigned dose $D = \rho T$. At the end of time T, N_1 of these cells are observed to be alive and transformed, N_2 are observed to be alive but not transformed and the remaining $N - (N_1+N_2)$ having died. In most of the published work, the empirical behavior of the quantities such as the surviving fraction $(N_1+N_2)/N$, the transformed fraction N_1/N, number transformed per surviving cell $N_1/(N_1+N_2)$, etc., are studied as a function of D or ρ. These quantities are studied in literature one at a time. What is desired, as was pointed out in [10], is to have a joint set of data for (N, N_1, N_2) made available for varying values of D, ρ and for different types of radiation, such as UV, gamma, neutron, etc. We have pleasantly learned recently through the courtesy of Dr. E. J. Ainsworth and Dr. T. C. H. Yang, both of Lawrence Berkeley Laboratory, that such data are indeed available. In fact, Dr. Yang has kindly agreed to provide us with at least some of the needed data.

Assuming that various cells are affected by the radiation independently of each other and that each acts in a similar manner independently of each other during the time $(0,T)$, given N, the conditional distribution of the vector $(N_1, N_2, N-N_1-N_2)$ will simply be a multinomial distribution with the needed formulas for the probabilities P(a cell is alive at T) and P(a cell is alive but not transformed at T) provided through our model. In particular, in the case of UV-radiation when the hypothesis $g(s) = s$ is valid, using the theory developed in [10] for our model, it can be shown that

P(a cell is alive at T)

$$= \exp[-(\frac{\delta}{\rho} + \frac{\pi_2 \theta}{\nu_1})D - \frac{\theta \rho \pi_1}{\nu_1} \frac{\gamma}{\alpha+\beta+\gamma} \psi(D,\rho)] \qquad (14)$$

and

P(a cell is alive but not transformed at T)

$$= P(a \text{ cell is alive at } T) \cdot \exp[-\frac{\theta \rho \pi_1}{\gamma_1} \frac{\beta}{\alpha+\beta+\gamma} \psi(D,\rho)] \qquad (15)$$

where

$$\psi(D,\rho) = \frac{D}{\rho} - \frac{1}{(\alpha+\beta+\gamma)} \{1 - \exp(-[\alpha+\beta+\gamma]\frac{D}{\rho})\}. \qquad (16)$$

The equations (14) and (15) in turn lead to the following interesting relation valid for all D.

$$\frac{\gamma}{\beta} \ln P(\text{cell is not transformed at } T \mid \text{alive at } T)$$

$$= \ln P(\text{cell is alive at } T) + [\frac{\delta}{\rho} + \frac{\theta \pi_2}{\nu_1}]D. \qquad (17)$$

Since the probabilities P(cell is not transformed at T | alive at T) and P(cell is alive at T) correspond to the empirical quantities $N_2/(N_1+N_2)$ and $(N_1+N_2)/N$ respectively, the relation (17), at least qualitatively, can be verified empirically for some appropriate constants $\frac{\gamma}{\beta}$ and $(\frac{\delta}{\rho} + \frac{\theta \pi_2}{\nu_1})$. The lack of support of (17), if so exhibited on the part of experimental data, would have to be interpreted as either that the hypothesis $g(s) = s$ is not valid or that the model itself needs some scrutiny as far as UV-radiation is concerned. This will have to be a subject of our future investigation.

5. Concluding Remarks.

(a) The present stochastic model is formulated in terms of hypothetical entities such as "primary" particles and clusters of "secondary" particles, each with certain hypothetical properties. The various formulas derived for the model involve two unspecified functions $g(\cdot)$ and $\delta(\rho)$ and a relatively large number of adjustable parameters namely, λ, α, β, γ, A, π_1 and $@_2$. The introduction of so many parameters was motivated by the desire not to omit a detail of the modeled phenomenon which might be important. Also, it is possible that in some cases certain apriori considerations may determine some of these parameters. For instance, the rate λ may be estimable through some physical experiments with no reference to the irradiated cells. Also for example, for the UV-radiation it may be considered appropriate to take $g(s) = s$ (see section 4). Such considerations in general will help reduce nonidentifiability of parameters if there is any. This, of course, will also depend upon the kind of data that are used to test the validity of our model.

(b) Again it would be of considerable interest to study the consistency of the present model with the empirical evidence available from the experiments in which the same total dose D is split into fractions, with each fraction of the dose D given after certain gaps in time. The reader may refer to Elkind, et al. [4] and Han and Elkind [6] for such experimental studies dealing with the effects of fractionated exposures on cells (see also a recent survey paper of Yang and Tobias [18]).

(c) It is often suggested (see Yang and Tobias [18]) that certain special types of misrepairs of the radiation induced damages may ultimately lead to cell transformations. Such finer details relating to the variety of possible repair mechanisms were intentionally kept to a minimum in our model in order to keep the model simple and yet useful. In this connection, the reader may refer to a recent paper of Tobias, et al [14] that was brought to the author's attention at this conference. This paper is primarily concerned with modeling the repair-misrepair aspect of the cell survival.

(d) Again the present model does not allow multiplication of the cells during the study period (0,T). This is not unreasonable for the case of high dose-rate where T is usually small. However for the case where the dose rate is small, T is generally large. In such a case multiplications of cells are possible. Consequently the present model would need an appropriate modification in order to allow such a possibility. This possibility is currently under investigation.

(e) It was pointed out at the conference that in general not all transformations are cancerous. Thus if we were to distinguish between the transformations that are cancerous and those that are not, instead of having only one risk for transformations through the rate β, we might consider the possibility of two separate risks, one for the repairable damage to become cancerous and another one for it to become transformed without becoming cancerous.

(f) Finally, assuming that $g(s) = s$ is valid in the case of UV-radiation, one may easily obtain from (14) the approximation

$$\ln P(a \text{ cell is alive at } T) \approx -\left(\frac{\delta}{\rho} + \frac{\theta \pi_2}{\nu_1}\right) D - \frac{\theta \pi_1 \gamma}{2\nu_1 \rho} D^2, \quad (18)$$

valid for small D and the approximation

$$\ln P(a \text{ cell is alive at } T) \approx \frac{\theta \rho \pi_1}{\nu_1} \frac{\gamma}{(\alpha+\beta+\gamma)^2}$$

$$-\left(\frac{\delta}{\rho} + \frac{\theta \pi_2}{\nu_1} + \frac{\theta \pi_1}{\nu_1} \frac{\gamma}{(\alpha+\beta+\gamma)}\right) D, \quad (19)$$

valid for large D. The reader may note the similarity between the expression (18) and the so called linear-quadratic dose-survival relationship based on the two-hit theory or the theory based on the double-strand breaks familiar to radiation biologists. For details of the latter theory we refer the reader to a recent book by Chadwick and Leenhouts [3].

6. Acknowledgements.

The author is grateful to Professor J. Neyman, Director, Statistical Laboratory, U. C., Berkeley, whose organization of an Interdisciplinary Cancer Study Conference at Berkeley provided the author an excellent opportunity for exchanging ideas with some eminent radiobiologists. In particular, the author was greatly benefited by the discussions he had at this conference with Drs. C. A. Tobias; E. J. Ainsworth and T. C. H. Yang, all from Lawrence Berkeley Laboratory.

7. References

[1] Barendsen, G. W. (1968) Responses of cultured cells, tumors and normal tissues of radiations of different linear energy transfer. *Curr. Top. Radiat. Res.* (ed. M. Ebert and A. Howard) 4, 293-356.

[2] Bedford, J. S., and Hall, E. J. (1963) Survival of HeLa cells cultured in vitro and exposed to protracted gamma-irradiation. *Int. J. Radiat. Biol.* 7 (4), 377-383.

[3] Chadwick, K. H., and Leenhouts, H. P. (1981) *The Molecular Theory of Radiation Biology*, Springer-Verlag, New York.

[4] Elkind, M. M., Sutton, H., and Moses, W. B. (1961) Postirradiation survival kinetics of mammalian cells grown in culture. *J. Cell. Comp. Physiol.* 58, Suppl. 1, 113-134.

[5] Hall, E. J., and Bedford, J. S. (1964) Dose rate: its effect on the survival of HeLa cells irradiated with gamma rays. *Radiat. Res.* 22, 305-315.

[6] Han, A., and Elkind, M. M. (1979) Transformation of mouse C3H/10T½ cells by single and fractionated doses of X-rays and fission-spectrum neutrons, *Cancer Res., 39*, 123-130.

[7] Han, A., Hill, C. K., and Elkind, M. M. (1980) Repair of cell killing and neoplastic transformation at reduced dose rates of ^{60}Co γ-rays, *Cancer Res., 40*, 3328-3332.

[8] Nauman, C. H., Underbrink, A. G., and Sparrow, A. H. (1975) Influence of radiation dose rate on somatic mutation induction in *Tradescantia* stamen hairs, *Radiat. Res. 62*, 79-96.

[9] Neyman, J. and Puri, P. S. (1976) A structural model of radiation effects in living cells. *Proc. Natn. Acad. Sci. U.S.A. 73*(10) 3360-3363.

[10] Neyman, J. and Puri, P. S. (1981) A hypothetical stochastic mechanism of radiation effects in single cells. *Proc. R. Soc. London.* Series B, *213*, 134-160.

[11] Payne, M. G. and Garrett, W. R. (1975) Models for cell survival with low LET radiation. *Radiat. Res. 62*, 169-179.

[12] Payne, M. G. and Garrett, W. R. (1975) Some relations between cell survival modelş having different inactivation mechanisms. *Radiat. Res. 62*, 388-394.

[13] Sparrow, A. H., Underbrink, A. G., and Rossi, H. H. (1972) Mutations induced in *Tradescantia* by small doses of X-rays and neutrons: analysis of dose-response curves. *Science. N. Y. 176*, 916-918.

[14] Tobias, C. S., Blakely, E. A., Ngo, F. Q. H., and Yang, T. C. H. (1980) The repair-misrepair model of cell survival. *Radiation Biology and Cancer Research.* (Ed: Meyn, A. and Withers, R.) 195-230, Raven Press, N. Y.

[15] Totter, J. R. (1972) Research programs of the Atomic Energy Commission's Division of Biology and Medicine relevant to problems of health and pollution. *Proc. Sixth Berkeley Symp. Math. Statist. and Prob. 6*, 71-100, Univ. Calif. Press, Berkeley.

[16] Upton, A. C., Randolph, M. L., Darden Jr., E. G., and Conklin, J. W. (1964) Relative biological effectiveness of fast neutrons for later somatic effects in mice. *Proc. Symp. Biological Effects of Neutron Irradiations, 2*, 337-347, International Atomic Energy Agency, Vienna.

[17] Upton, A. C., Randolph, M. L., and Conklin, J. W. (1967) Late effects of fast neutrons and gamma rays in mice as influenced by the dose rate irradiation: life shortening. *Radiat. Res. 32*, 493-509.

[18] Yang, T. C. H., and Tobias, C. A. (1980) Radiation and cell transformation *in vitro*. *Adv. Biological and Med. Physics. 17*, 417-461.

Studies on the Survival Frequencies of Irradiated Mammalian Cells with and without Cancer Cell Morphology

Tracy Chui-hsu Yang and Cornelius A. Tobias

Division of Biology and Medicine
Lawrence Berkeley Laboratory
and
Department of Biophysics and Medical Physics
University of California
Berkeley, California

1. Introduction

X-rays, which are an ionizing radiation, were discovered by Wilhelm C. Roentgen in 1895. Shortly after his discovery, many physicians began to apply radiation to cancer treatment. Swedish physicians, Drs. J. T. Stënbeck and T. A. V. Sjogren, first claimed that radiation cured a skin tumor on a patient's nose in 1899 (1). Soon afterwards, however, the potential carcinogenic effect of radiation was noticed because many radiologists began to develop skin ulceration and skin tumors on their left hands, which were X-rayed (2). Perhaps the most clear evidence that ionizing radiation can be carcinogenic to humans is the data obtained on the cancer incidence in atomic bomb survivors at Hiroshima and Nagasaki. The incidence of cancer was significantly higher among those survivors closest to the explosion, and decreased with distance from the center (3). Over the past several decades, numerous animal experiments with radiation have been performed, and the results show a strong dependence on dose in cancer induction. Within a relatively low dose range, the frequency of many types of cancer generally increases with dose (4).

Although there appears to be a strong correlation between radiation and cancer induction in animals, the role of radiation in carcinogenesis is not yet completely understood. The biological complexity of the animal system and the presence of various kinds of chemical and biological carcinogens in the environment make it very difficult to determine whether the observed high incidence of tumors in irradiated animals is the direct result of radiation or a consequence of the interaction between radiation and other carcinogen(s). A simpler model system is needed in order to answer this fundamental question of radiobiology, i.e., whether radiation acts as an oncogen (an initiator) or as a cocarcinogen (a promoter).

Cultured mammalian cells have been used over the past twenty years as a model system for studying the mechanism(s) of cancer formation at the molecular and cellular level. Using cell culture techniques, the interaction between radiation and oncogenic viruses has been investigated, and a viral enhancement of the frequency of neoplastic cell transformation (i.e., the frequency of normal cells changing into cancer cells) has been commonly observed (5,6). The effects of radiation on chemical carcinogens in inducing neoplastic cell transformation are less well studied. Synergistic effects occur when the frequency of cell transformation as a result of the combined treatment of both agents is greater than the sum of the frequency of cell transformation for each agent. These synergistic effects have been found when a proper sequence of treatment with X-rays and benzo(a)pyrene was used (7). Radiation, therefore, can act as cocarcinogen for many other types of oncogens.

This report will focus on the carcinogenic effects of ionizing radiation in mammalian cells. Cell culture techniques and the cell systems commonly used for studying the carcinogenic effects of ionizing radiation will be described. We will also discuss our results on cell survival and on neoplastic cell transformation using low- and high-LET radiation. (LET = linear energy transfer: the rate of energy dissipation along the track of the ionizing particle. The unit generally used is kilovolts per micrometer of tissue, keV/μm.) Finally, there will be a brief discussion on the possible mechanism(s) of action of radiation in carcinogenesis.

2. Cell Systems and Methods Used for Studying Radiation-induced Cancer

2.1. Cell System

Both primary cultures and cell lines have been used to study the radiation induction of neoplastic cell transformation in vitro. In general, primary cultured cells can be obtained using mechanical and enzymatic methods to dissociate the normal animal tissue into single cells, which can then be grown for many weeks at 37°C in media containing proper nutrients. Because the primary cultured cells are taken directly from normal tissue and they maintain the characteristics of normal cells, many investigators have chosen them for studying cell transformation in vitro. In fact, the first cell experiment which demonstrated clearly that ionizing radiation may act as a carcinogen was done with short-term primary cultures from midterm golden hamster embryos (8).

Because of their uniformity in response to radiation and because of their high-plating efficiency and handling ease, established cell lines have been widely used by radiation biophysicists to study cellular responses to radiation. The most popular cell line that has been used for investigating radiation-induced neoplastic cell transformation is the C3H10T½, which was established by Reznikoff et al. in 1973 (9). Embryo cells from the C3H mouse were grown in dishes for many passages through the cell cycle, and then cloned. One of the cloned cells (clone 8) showed a high sensitivity of postconfluent inhibition of cell division, and this clone was selected subsequently to study the chemical carcinogen-induced neoplastic cell transformation in vitro. In nonconfluent or sparse cultures, cells are fibroblast-like with long cytoplasmic process. Once they reach a confluent stage, the cells form a flat even monolayer and appear somewhat epithelial.

2.2. General Method for Quantitative Determination of Neoplastic Cell Transformation in Vitro

A schematic diagram showing the general method, which we have used to determine the survival frequency of cells and the frequency of radiation-induced neoplastic cell transformation, is given in Figure 1.

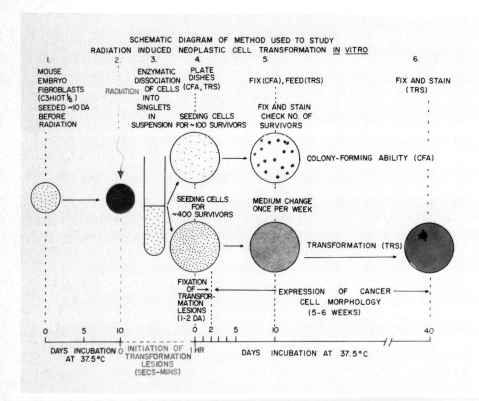

Figure 1. A schematic diagram showing the experimental method used for studying neoplastic cell transformation of C3H10T½ cells induced by ionizing radiation.

Cells from stock culture were plated into 35-mm tissue culture dishes containing 3 ml growth medium (BME with 10% calf serum) and incubated at 37 °C for about 10 days. At the end of the incubation period, the cells formed an even confluent monolayer and remained in the G1 phase of the cell cycle. These cells were then exposed to various doses of radiation. Immediately after the irradiation, the cells were treated with a solution of trypsin-EDTA and dissociated into singlets in suspension.

For each radiation experiment, two sets of 100-mm tissue culture dishes were prepared, one set to determine the percentage of survival and another set to check the number of foci showing cancer cell morphology. The same population of cells received a given radiation dose; therefore, the same population was used to determine both the cell survival and the frequency of neoplastic cell transformation. For each radiation dose, at least four dishes were seeded with cells which would give about 100 survivors in each dish after 10 to 12 days of incubation at 37 °C. After the cells were fixed with glutaldehyde and stained with methylene blue, the colonies that contained more than fifty cells were scored as survivors.

Because the frequency of radiation-induced neoplastic cell transformation is very low, a large number of cells and dishes were needed. In general, about 30 to 50 dishes were used for low doses and 15 to 20 dishes for high doses; each dish was plated with cells that would yield about 400 survivors. After irradiation, the cells were incubated for 5 to 6 weeks at 37 °C with a medium change once per week. At the end of this period the cells were fixed and stained to see the number of transformed foci. The criteria for scoring transformed foci for C3H10T½ cells have been described in detail by Reznikoff et al. (10). Both type II, a focus showing massive piling up of cells into virtually opaque multilayers without pronounced criss-crossing, and type III, a focus composed of highly polar, fibroblastic, multilayered criss-crossed arrays of densely stained cells, were scored as transformed foci in our studies. Transformed foci can be easily recognized, since they are dense and discrete, in contrast with the flat background of control cells (Figure 2).

Once we knew the number of cells seeded, the percentage of survival, and the number of transformed foci, we could calculate the frequency of neoplastic cell transformation per survivor for a given radiation dose.

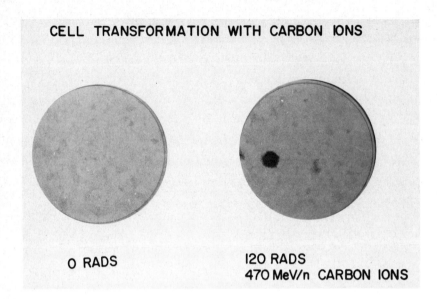

Figure 2. A comparison between a control dish containing evenly spread monolayer C3H10T½ cells with no transformed colonies and a dish showing a discrete and dense neoplastic transformed focus in cells irradiated with 120 rad neon ions.

3. Quantitative Results of Radiation Studies

The unique heavy-ion radiation facilities at Lawrence Berkeley Laboratory (LBL) make possible the studies on the effects of energetic high-LET radiation on cell inactivation and on neoplastic cell transformation. Because heavy-ion radiation gives a better depth-dose distribution in tissue, a lower oxygen effect, a higher relative biological effectiveness (RBE) in killing tumor cells, and a smaller cell age effect than X-rays and gamma rays, a program to study the potential usefulness of heavy-ion radiation in treating human cancer has been initiated and is in progress at LBL (11). As one part of the Biology and Medicine heavy-ion radiation program, we are systematically investigating the potential carcinogenic and mutagenic effects of low- and high-LET radiation at the cellular level. From these studies, we anticipate additional insight into the molecular and cellular mechanisms of radiation carcinogenesis which will provide quantitative information useful for assessing the undesirable biological effects of cosmic rays in space. Some of our recent experimental results are presented here.

Figure 3 shows the dose-response curves for cells irradiated either with X-rays or with 13.2 MeV/n (million electron volts per nucleon) carbon ions accelerated at 88-inch cyclotron at LBL.

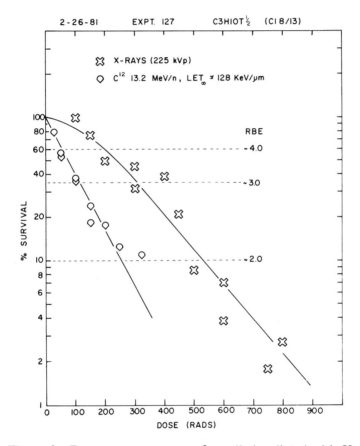

Figure 3. Dose-response curves for cells irradiated with X-rays or 13.2 MeV/n carbon ions. RBE values (the ratio of the X-ray dose and the carbon-ion dose for an equal biological effect) are given at different survival levels.

For X-irradiated cells, the survival curve shows a significant shoulder with an extrapolation number (n) of about 2, which was determined by extrapolating the exponential portion of the survival curve back to zero dose. The survival curve for cells irradiated with 13.2 MeV/n carbon ions (LET $\approx$ 128 keV/μm) appears to be a simple exponential one. For a given lethal effect, carbon particles are more effective than X-rays. In order to kill 90% cells, for example, it takes less than 300 rad of carbon ions, which is about half the dose of X-rays. The relative biological effectiveness (RBE) for carbon ions at 90% cell killing, or 10% survival, is, therefore, about 2.0. The RBE value for carbon ions varies with the level of cell killing: it increases with a decrease in cell killing.

The effects of ionizing radiation on neoplastic cell transformation is shown in Figure 4. The number of transformants per survivor is plotted as a function of radiation dose on a semi-log scale. Both X-rays and carbon ions can induce neoplastic cell transformation. The frequency of cell transformation per survivor increases with radiation dose and appears to reach a plateau at about 600 rad for X-rays. For a given dose, 13.2 MeV/n carbon particles show a greater effect than X-rays in inducing neoplastic cell transformation, since the number of transformants per survivor for all the carbon-ion doses used are consistently above the curve for X-rays. The same experimental data are plotted also on a linear scale in Figure 5. The RBE value for carbon particles varies with the dose level, from about 1.9 at relative high dose to about 3.0 for low doses. High-LET heavy ion radiation, i.e., carbon ions with LET $\approx$ 128 keV/μm, therefore, can cause cell killing and neoplastic cell transformation more effectively than X-rays.

However, when the frequency of transformation is compared on an equal survival level, no significant difference between these two different modalities of radiation has been seen. Figure 6 shows a plot of the number of transformants per survival as a function of the log of percent of survival, and the dose-response curve appears to be curvilinear.

Some of the transformation lesions induced by X-rays are repairable. When X-irradiated confluent C3H10T½ cells were incubated for 24 hours at 37°C before being plated into dishes as singlets, the transformation frequency decreased significantly. The results of an experiment designed to study the repair kinetics of transformation lesions in confluent cells are given in Figure 7. For both radiation doses used, 600 and 300 rad, there is

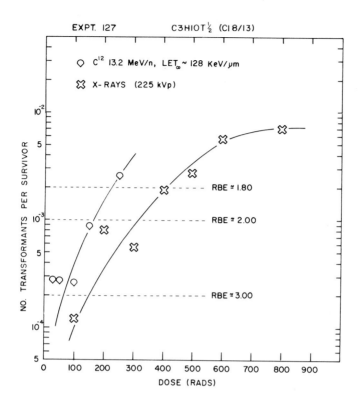

Figure 4. Effects of ionizing radiation on neoplastic cell transformation. At equal doses, the number of transformants per survivor for carbon ions is consistently higher than that for X-rays. The RBE values for various frequencies of transformation are given.

clearly a significant decrease of transformation frequency with a 24-hour period. Cells irradiated with 600 rad, for example, showed a decrease in the number of transformants per survivor from about 3×10^{-3} to about 7×10^{-4}. The number of transformants per survivor for a single dose 300 rad is about 7×10^{-4}, which suggests that about half of the transformation

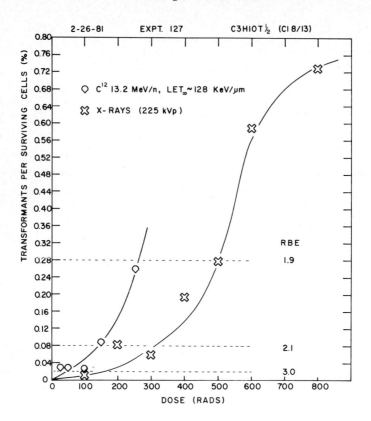

Figure 5. A linear plot of the percent of transformants per survivor as a function of radiation dose for X-rays and carbon particles.

lesions induced by 600 rad X-rays are repairable. The number of transformation lesions remaining in cells appears to diminish exponentially with incubation time, although present data are not precise enough to make a

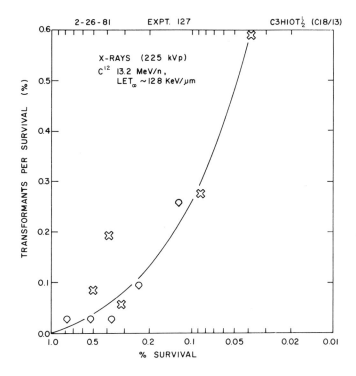

Figure 6. The percent of transformants per survival is plotted as a function of percent of survival. A curvilinear curve appears to fit both the X ray and the carbon-ion data reasonably well. (XBL 815-9844)

determination on the repair rate.

4. Possible Mechanisms of Radiation Carcinogenesis

Our experimental results show that for a given dose, energetic carbon ions with a high LET can be more effective than X-rays in causing both cell killing and neoplastic cell transformation. The high efficiency with which heavy ions produce these two important biological effects may be a result of their unique physical properties. As a heavy particle passes through water, an energy transfer from the heavy ion to the water molecules occurs because of the physical interactions. One result of this energy transfer is the ionization of water molecules which then form free

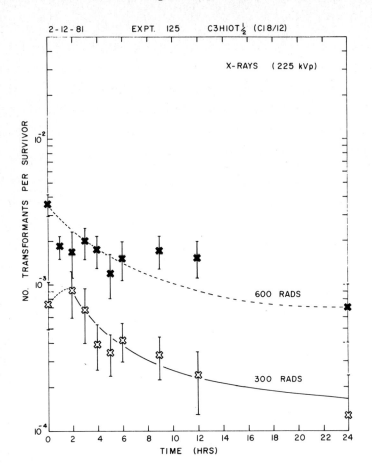

Figure 7. The repair kinetics of transformation lesions in confluent C3H10T½ cells irradiated with two different doses of X-rays. (XBL 815-9901)

radicals through chemical reactions. Thus, a dense ionization track will form along the trajectory of a moving heavy ion. In general, the size of the track increases with the energy of the heavy particle, and a microdosimetric structure of heavy-ion tracks in tissue has been proposed (12).

The ionization track has two regions: the core and the penumbra. The core is a narrow central zone with a radius in water much less than one micrometer in which half the total energy of the heavy ion is deposited through physical processes of excitation and electron plasma oscillations. The penumbra is a spherical zone that surrounds the core; energy deposition in the penumbra occurs mainly in ionization events of secondary electrons released by the primary particle at the center of the core. The local energy density in the core is very high and decreases with the square of increasing radius in the penumbra. Figure 8 shows the size of an ionization track for a 10 MeV/n heavy particle.

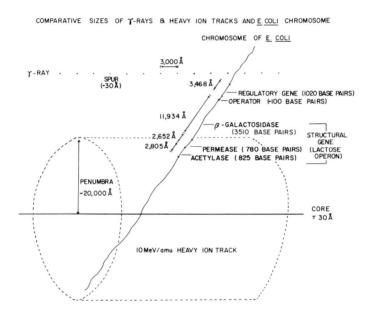

Figure 8. An ionization track of a 10 MeV/n heavy particle and the track of a photon of X-rays are compared with part of an *E. coli* chromosome. Notice the large size of the heavy ion track penumbra.

If this heavy ion hits a DNA molecule perpendicularly, the maximum number of base pairs that can be affected is about 9 by the core, and about 10,000 by the penumbra. Therefore, a single heavy ion can make a cluster of damage in several genes that are in a linear sequence. Unlike heavy-ion radiation, X rays only produce sparse ionization, and the average distance between two ionizing centers (spurs) can be about 3,000 Å. Thus, in a microvolume, heavy ions can produce a much higher density of ionization than X-rays, and consequently heavy-ion radiation can induce a greater number of lesions within a given region than X-rays. This high density of lesions may enhance the probability for interaction between lesions and may interfere with the enzymatic repair processes in the cell. As a result, there will be a greater number of misrepaired lesions in heavy-ion irradiated cells than in X-irradiated ones. Misrepaired lesions can cause cell killing or neoplastic cell transformation, as proposed by the repair-misrepair model (13).

In irradiated mammalian cells, various types of lesions in the cell nucleus have been observed, including single DNA strand breaks, double DNA strand breaks, base damage, and DNA and nuclear protein cross-links. Shortly after irradiation, these lesions will be either repaired perfectly (eurepair) or repaired incorrectly (misrepair). A simplified diagram showing the possible pathway of lesions in irradiated mammalian cells is given in Figure 9. Cells with no misrepaired lesions will survive the radiation assault and remain normal. Misrepaired lesions can be lethal or nonlethal to cells. Cells containing nonlethal misrepaired lesions will become mutated and/or neoplastic transformed ones; cells possessing lethal misrepaired lesions will die. Ionizing radiation appears to be much more effective in producing a lethal lesion than causing mutation and neoplastic transformation in mammalian cells. A dose 600 rad of X-rays, for instance, will kill about 90% C3H10T½ cells, while of the survivors less than 1% will be transformed and 0.1% will be mutated. This apparent difference in response to radiation may relate to the difference in the target size for cell killing, mutation, and neoplastic transformation.

When the transformation frequency per survivor for low- and high-LET radiation is compared at an equal survival level, the experimental data show that there is no significant difference (Figure 6). This result seems to suggest that a constant portion of nonlethal lesions may be responsible for the cell transformation. If a linear plot of the transformation frequency per survivor versus the percentage of survival is calculated, however, a curvilinear response is found, as shown in Figure 10. At high cell-killing level, radiation appears to form more transformation lesions per survivor. The

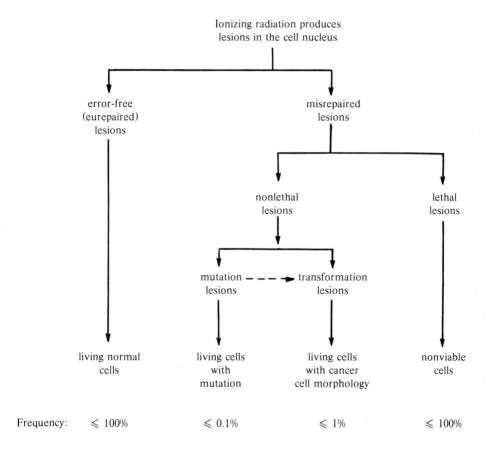

Figure 9. A diagram showing the possible pathways of primary lesions induced by ionizing radiation in the mammalian cells. The maximum frequency for various biological effects of ionizing radiation is given under each column.

transformation lesion, therefore, is not a constant portion of nonlethal lesions for different doses. One of the possible implications of this result is that a higher proportion of lesions becomes misrepaired nonlethal lesions at high doses than low doses. Because interaction between lesions

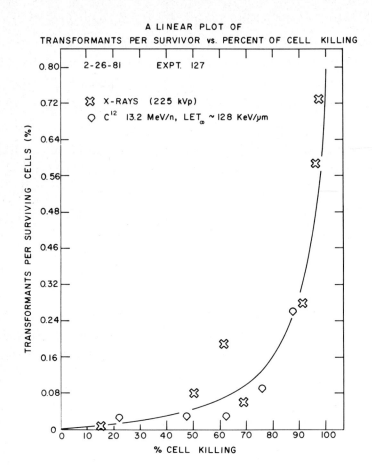

Figure 10. A linear plot of percent of transformants per survivor as a function of percent of cell killing.

produced by different heavy particles or photons becomes more probable at high doses, some of the transformation lesions may be a result of error-prone interactions between primary lesions.

It has been assumed that mammalian cell nuclear DNA is the primary target for cell killing by low and moderately high doses of ionization radiation. There is also some evidence to suggest that DNA is an important target for radiation-induced neoplastic cell transformation. Studies with isotope-labelled nucleotides, for example, show that tritiated thymidine can cause neoplastic cell transformation in vitro (14). Moreover, it was found that cells exposed to 5-bromodeoxyuridine (a DNA analog) before X-irradiation gave a frequency of cell transformation several times higher than cells treated with radiation alone. The concentration of the DNA analog used was about 10^{-5} M, which did not cause a significant number of cells to transform (15).

Ionizing radiation can be mutagenic to mammalian cells. A common genetic marker used extensively for studying radiation mutagenesis in mammalian cells is the 6-thioguanine resistant DNA analog. Normal cells are extremely sensitive to this DNA analog and are usually killed when they are incubated with a growth medium containing 6-thioguanine at a concentration of 5 μg/ml. After radiation treatment, however, a small fraction of cells can survive in the 6-thioguanine medium because of a gene mutation on the X chromosome. We studied the mutagenecity of heavy-ion radiation and found that high-LET neon particles (425 MeV/n; 32 keV/μm) are many times more effective than X-rays in inducing the 6-thioguanine resistant mutants, as shown in Figure 11. Since heavy ions are more effective than X-rays in producing both the neoplastic cell transformation and the 6-thioguanine mutation, there is a possibility that this type of mutation lesion (a deletion and rearrangement) may be involved in ionizing radiation-induced neoplastic cell transformation. The precise relationship between these two types of lesions, however, is unclear at present.

Mechanisms other than a point mutation, e.g., a frameshift mutation or a small deletion, have been suggested for neoplastic transformation. Mutation at the chromosome level, e.g., aneuploidy due to nondisjunction, has been proposed for the diethylstilbestrol-induced neoplastic transformation (16). Ionizing radiation is known to cause chromosome aberrations effectively. It seems plausible that some macrochromosomal aberrations may be related to the neoplastic transformation lesions. More than one type of DNA lesions, therefore, may contribute to the radiation-induced neoplastic cell transformation. The fact that there are repairable and non-repairable transformation lesions, as shown by the results of repair kinetics

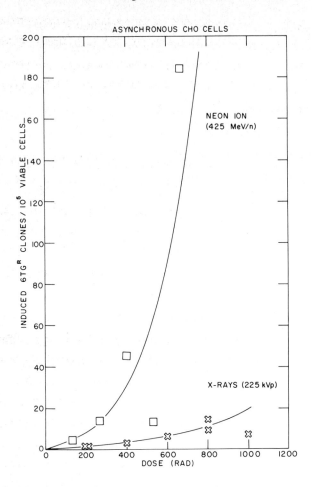

Figure 11. A comparison between the mutagenicity of X-rays and neon ions. The 6-thioguanine resistant was used as the genetic marker. Mutants were selected by growing irradiated asynchronous Chinese hamster ovary cells in medium containing 5 μg/ml 6-thioguanine for two weeks at 37 °C.

study (Figure 7), tends to support this idea.

The frequency of neoplastic cell transformation by ionizing radiation is generally less than 1%, which suggests that in mammalian cells the transformation target may be 100 times smaller than that for cell killing. The transformation target probably consists of many genes in the cell.

How these transformation genes are distributed among the chromosomes and what are the DNA sequences of these genes are two important questions to be answered in the future.

The development of cancer in animals exposed to ionizing radiation can be a complicated and long-term process. The possible mechanism of action of radiation-induced carcinogenesis is briefly presented in Figure 12. In the cell nucleus, within a second of radiation exposure, various free radicals are formed and will react with important biological macromolecules, e.g., DNA or chromosome proteins, to produce many types of lesions. Within minutes to hours, lesions will be either correctly repaired or misrepaired through enzymatic and nonenzymatic processes. An alteration of DNA or nuclear protein or both due to misrepair can cause some genetic and epigenetic effects. These effects may directly (or indirectly through an activation of viral information) initiate the neoplastic cell transformation. After weeks of proliferation, cells with transformation lesions express properties of cancer cells. Some transformed cells will be selected by various physiological and immunological factors to develop into a cancer. Consequently, the entire process of cancer development in animals may take many years.

At present our studies on cell transformation in vitro are designed primarily to investigate the molecular and cellular events that occur in cells within hours to days after irradiation. Most of our efforts are focused on understanding the mechanisms of initiation of carcinogenesis. The cell system, however, can also be very useful for studying the phenomenon of genetic expression. With further improvement and development of techniques, it may become possible to conduct experiments in vitro to study factors that can affect the selection process. Complementary to the animal work, the in vitro neoplastic cell transformation study with radiation may help us to interpret the radiation carcinogenesis in animals correctly and to understand the dynamic process and mechanisms of cancer formation in man.

Possible Mechanisms of Action of Radiation-induced Carcinogenesis

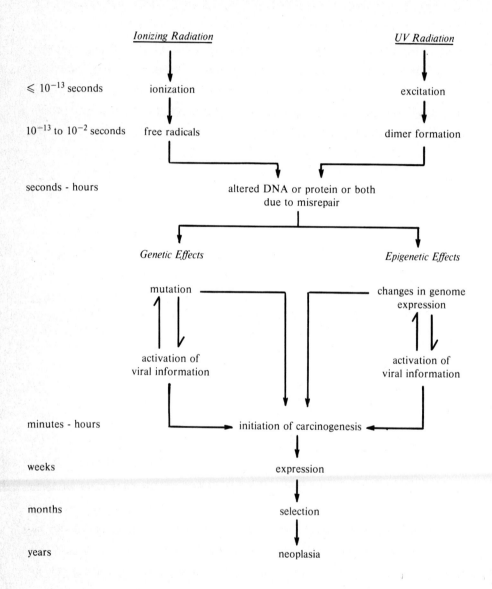

Figure 12. A simplified diagram showing the possible mechanisms of action of radiation in carcinogenesis. The time scale is provided only for an approximation.

5. Acknowledgements

We would like to acknowledge the excellent technical help from F. Abrams, L. Craise, C. Perez, and D. Tse and to thank M. Pirruccello for editorial assistance. The encouragement and interest in this work by Drs. E. L. Alpen and E. J. Ainsworth are deeply appreciated. The C3H10T½ cells were kindly provided by Drs. C. Heidelberger and S. Mondel. These studies were supported by NASA, the National Cancer Institute (Grant No. CA15184), and the Office of Health and Environmental Research of the U. S. Department of Energy under Contract W-7405-ENG-48.

6. References

1. Cassarett, A. P. 1968. *Radiation Biology*, pp. 2-3. Englewood Cliffs, New Jersey: Prentice-Hall, Inc.

2. Upton, A. C. 1969. *Radiation Injury*, pp. 57-60. Chicago, Illinois: University of Chicago.

3. National Academy of Sciences. 1980. *The Effects on Population of Exposure to Low Levels of Ionizing Radiation: 1980*, p. 189. Washington, D. C.: National Academy Press.

4. Walburg, H. E. Jr. 1974. Experimental radiation carcinogenesis. *Advances in Radiation Biology 4*, 209-254.

5. Pollock, E. and G. Todaro. 1968. Radiation enhancement of SV40 transformation in 3T3 and human cells. *Nature (London) 219*, 520-521.

6. Yang, T. C. H., C. A. Tobias, E. A. Blakely, L. M. Craise, I. S. Madfes, C. Perez, and J. Howard. 1980. Enhancement effects of high-energy neon particles on the viral transformation of mouse C3H10T½ cells in vitro. *Radiat. Res. 81*, 208-223.

7. DiPaolo, J. A., P. J. Donovan, and N. C. Popesou. 1976. Kinetics of Syrian hamster cells during x-irradiation enhancement of transformation in vitro by chemical carcinogen. *Radiat. Res. 66*, 310-325.

8. Borek, C. and L. Sachs. 1968. In vitro cell transformation by x-irradiation. *Nature (London) 210*, 276-278.

9. Reznikoff, C. A., D. W. Brankov, and C. Heidelberger. 1973. Establishment and characteristics of a cloned line of C3H mouse embryo cells sensitive to postconfluence inhibition of division. *Cancer Res. 33*, 3231-3238.

10. Reznikoff, C. A., J. S. Betram, D. W. Brankov, and C. Heidelberger. 1973. Quantitative and qualitative studies of chemical transformation of cloned C3H mouse embryo cells sensitive to postconfluence inhibition of cell division. *Cancer Res. 33*, 3239-3249.

11. Pirruccello, M. C. and C. A. Tobias, eds. 1980. *Biological and Medical Research with Accelerated Heavy Ions at the Bevalac, 1977-1980.* Lawrence Berkeley Laboratory Report LBL-11220.

12. Chatterjee, A. and H. J. Chaefer. 1976. Microdosimetric structure of heavy ion tracks in tissue. *Radiat. Environm. Biophys. 13*, 215-227.

13. Tobias, C. A., E. A. Blakely, F. Q. H. Ngo, and T. C. H. Yang. 1980. The repair-misrepair model of cell survival. *Radiation Biology in Cancer Research* (R. E. Meyn and H. R. Withers, eds.), pp 195-230. New York: Raven Press.

14. LeMotte, P. K., S. J. Adelstein, and J. B. Little. 1978. Transformation of mouse embryo fibroblasts (10T½) with incorporated radioisotopes. *Radiat. Res. 74*, 537. (Abstract).

15. Little, J. B. 1977. Radiation carcinogenesis in vitro: Implication for mechanisms. *Origins of Human Cancer (B)* (H. H. Hiatt, J. D. Watson, and J. A. Winsten, eds.), pp 923-939. New York: Cold Spring Harbor Laboratory.

16. Barrett, J. C., A. Wong, and J. A. McLachlan. 1981. Diethylstilbestrol induces neoplastic transformation without measurable gene mutation at two loci. *Science 212*, 1402-1404.

Some Remarks on Cancer as a State of Disorganization at the Cellular and Supracellular Levels

H. Rubin

Department of Molecular Biology
University of California
Berkeley, California 94720

It has become the custom, well attested in this meeting, to consider cancer as a disease of cells, or more specifically of a single cell which has multiplied to form a tumor. It is assumed there is a molecular lesion -- is there any choice? -- in the form of a change in the base sequence or arrangement of DNA, or the expression of a virus. Even the so called epigenetic theories, which invoke a change in the non-genetic material of the cell, assume a change in chemical composition of some discrete molecule or species of molecule in the cell. It is on this basis that statistical models of the origin, growth and metastasis are built. I wish to present evidence that this type of molecular -- or even cellular -- thinking is inadequate and may be quite misleading for comprehending the problem of carcinogenesis. I have covered some of this ground in a guest editorial in the Journal of the National Cancer Institute (1), and I refer you there for references, but I will go somewhat beyond the materials and ideas covered there.

Unlike microorganisms, cells from multicellular organisms and explicitly for our purposes those of vertebrates, behave differently when they are growing as isolated single cells, or in small groups, or in large groups such as characterize a tissue. There are many examples of this dependence on population density and size in tissue culture studies and in the development of the organism. One example is the development of the nervous system in the chick. A standard sized piece of the chick primitive streak blastoderm produces nervous tissue when placed on the chick chorioallantoic membrane (2). One-sixteenth of this piece never produces nervous tissue, although it contains large numbers of cells and remains viable. But 16 such small pieces fused into a single mass do produce nervous tissue. If they are placed in a dispersed cluster, they fail to produce nervous tissue. There is a level of organization higher than that of the cell which is required to allow the cell and its neighbors to express their potential for normal development.

Once the developmental potential of the cell has been expressed, i.e., it is fully differentiated, that particular state is stably inherited. All the offspring of a liver cell will be liver cells and all the offspring of a basal cell of the epidermis will give rise to skin, despite the fact that the nuclear DNA of cells from different tissues (with the exception of cells of the immune system) have the same base sequence in their DNA. How this stable differentiated state is brought about and maintained is unknown -- one of the great mysteries of life.

There is one way to change the differentiated state of a cell, and that is to separate it from its neighbors in a procedure called cell culture. There most epithelial cells quickly lose some of their differentiated functions and indeed, I know of no case where the full and balanced differentiated potential of an epithelial tissue has been maintained for long in dispersed cell culture (3). If, after a few divisions, the cells are packed together in a large mass, they may regain their original capacities, but after a while even this tactic fails. The cells have undergone some irreversible shift in their potential. What we see here is the importance of the organized state of a tissue in maintaining the differentiated state.

An apparent exception to this behavior is the typical connective tissue cell called the fibroblast. Fibroblasts can be maintained for many generations in culture, and indeed cell lines can be derived which can be maintained indefinitely in culture. It is not so surprising that epithelial and fibroblastic cells should behave in a disparate manner as the epithelial cells are maintained in a tight, fixed relation to each other in the organism while the fibroblasts are only loosely associated, and keep moving around. Thus being dispersed is not as big a change in life style for the fibroblast as it is for the epithelial cell. There is a hitch though even with the fibroblasts. They also change in culture, though in a more subtle way than the epithelial cells. Their growth rate gradually slows down with repeated transfers. If they are human fibroblasts they eventually stop growing, unless they were cancer cells in the first place (4). If they were mouse cells, they also gradually lose their growth potential but they reach a crisis point at which they either die out, like human cells, or they start growing faster and become adapted to cell culture (5). When they do that, they are called a cell line, and they are very different in their properties from normal fibroblasts. For example, they look different, have a different number of chromosomes, and display different growth behavior. If they are injected back into the animal, they usually produce cancer. The point I am getting at is that from the day that the fibroblasts are separated from each other and placed in a foreign environment, they start to undergo irreversible changes. These may lead to the loss of growth potential (a loss euphemistically called senescence) or to acquisition of a relatively stable capacity to grow in culture and produce tumors in animals. These changes occur in the absence of chemical or physical carcinogens. Just as it was necessary to have cells in the presence of their neighbors to permit differentiation to occur, it is necessary to maintain this relationship in order to perpetuate the differentiated state.

An interesting example of the relevance of these observations to carcinogenesis was provided a few years ago by Dr. DeOme, the founder of our Cancer Research Laboratory. He was working with a strain of mice which had a high incidence of breast cancer, but overt hyperplastic nodules and tumors only developed after a period of 8 or 9 months (6). If he removed the mammary gland tissue, dispersed the cells, and injected them back into gland-free fat pads, overt growths developed within 2 months. If he transplanted pieces of intact mammary gland he did not get this effect. The simple act of disorganizing the tissue greatly accelerated the onset of the tumors.

The importance of organization in maintaining the normal state, and in producing the malignant state can be illustrated by another case. If germinal tissue from the ovary or testes of a mouse is placed in a foreign site in the body, a cancer called a teratocarcinoma frequently develops. This is a particularly gruesome cancer because it can produce all the different tissues of the body, but not in the form of complete organs and not in their normal relationship to one another. All the different tissues are generated from "stem cells" which have the undifferentiated appearance of highly malignant cells. If some of these carcinoma stem cells are injected into a normal mouse embryo at a very early stage of development, the embryo will go on to develop into an adult mouse in a perfectly normal way (7). What is more, many of its perfectly normal tissues are derived from the injected cancer cells, and there is no sign of a tumor. By being placed in an environment in which cells have a strong mutual interaction that leads to normal development, the cancer cells are regimented in such a way as to reacquire their normal developmental potential.

Another example will be instructive in showing the importance of supracellular organization in cancer. Certain parts of a newt can regenerate after the part has been cut off and other parts cannot. Cancer can be produced in either of these regions by injecting a chemical carcinogen under the skin (8). If the cancer is produced in a strongly regenerating region of the animal, it will almost always regress. If it is in a weakly regenerating region it will almost invariably become invasive and kill the animal. Again it appears that the presence of a strong developmental field can reverse the malignant process. These examples also indicate that the malignant process is not, in these cases at least, an irreversible process as one would expect it to be if it were caused by a change in the chemical composition or the arrangement of the DNA in the cell.

We tend to think of the malignant transformation of cells as a rare event at the cellular level. And indeed, it must be a rare event in the body. If it occurred with the frequency of mutations, i.e., a probability of $\sim 10^{-6}$ per cell division, and considering we have ca. 10^{14} cells in our body, many of them actively dividing, we should be developing hundreds of thousands or millions of incipient new malignancies every day. Indeed, we should never be born without being full of tumors. When we examine small numbers of cells in culture the picture is even more disturbing. Dr. Yang, in his interesting presentation told us that one transformed focus is formed within 6 weeks for every 10^5 cells seeded of the $C3H10T^{1/2}$ line he uses to assay the carcinogenic activity of x-rays (9). Radiation increases the frequency of transformation to 1 in 100 of the survivors of the radiation. The frequency of transformation is very much dependent on the population density at which the irradiated cells are seeded, with the frequency being much higher when the cells are seeded at low rather than high density. Dr. Tobias indicated that even among the non-transformed survivors of radiation, there is a good chance that many, if not most of them, are altered in some way not detected by direct observation. This is reminiscent of the results obtained in Heidelberger's laboratory with chemical carcinogenesis (10). When single cells were treated with 3-methylcholanthrene, and then grown to a heavily populated culture, up to 100% of the cells were either transformed or produced colonies which had transformed cells. Yet, this carcinogen as well as others must be repeatedly applied to tissues of the intact organism before it produces a tumor, despite the fact that millions of cells are exposed at each application. We must conclude that the state of organization of cells in a tissue in the intact organism has much to do with the fortunate fact that the quantitative results of cell transformation in tissue culture cannot be translated into the degree of risk in the whole organism. Indeed, it has been speculated that cells in culture are 10^{10} times more likely to undergo transformation than are cells in the animal if the latter is measured by appearance of a tumor (11).

I bring these considerations to your attention because they are often ignored in discussions of carcinogenesis, and I believe they must be included in any analysis of the mechanisms involved. They show that animal cells cannot be adequately described by models obtained from microorganisms. The state of organization of animal cells plays a dominant role in their behavior, and any disruption of that organized state radically alters that behavior. The organized behavior of animal cells is altered during differentiation in a hereditary way which does not involve irreversible changes in the DNA (12), and that alteration depends itself on the preexisting organization of the cells. Malignancy can be considered a state of disorganization of a tissue, and it probably reflects a level of disorganization within the cell (13). There is no more reason to believe that the disorganization requires a somatic mutation than there is to believe that differentiation of most tissues requires a change in the nucleotide sequence of DNA. That is not to say that a mutation cannot induce transformation, only that other mechanisms for which there are no models in microorganisms have to be considered. Indeed, a leading proponent of the somatic mutation hypothesis of cancer has largely abandoned that model for the origin of human cancer, although he has proposed one which involves transposition of the genetic material (14). I subscribe that we must consider cancer as basically a developmental problem involving the organization of the cell, and the organization of cells in groups. While the genetic material of the cell cannot be excluded from such a consideration, it should be considered in the context of the cell as a whole, and of the tissue in which the cell functions. In that context, the genetic material is as much under direction of the cell as it is the director of the cell. I suspect our understanding of the malignant transformation will parallel our understanding of the mechanism of differentiation.

We have tended to look upon the malignant transformation of cells as an all or none phenomenon. This probably results from our search for simplification and for systems which provide relatively simple answers. For example, some viruses which are popularly used in cancer research produce a sharp change to malignancy within a day after infection. But a consideration in depth of the natural history of cancer in man and rodents shows that cancer rarely if ever happens in this way. There are strong indications that the process has been going on for years before a tumor becomes detectable (13). And after it becomes detectable the tumor usually proceeds through several stages which may be successive or alternative, but the end result is a higher *degree* of malignancy. This process is called progression, and it is central to the understanding of malignancy. Yet this central aspect of malignancy is obliterated by the simplifying models we have made for our own convenience in the laboratory, and this is particularly true for viral carcinogenesis, where I have played a part in creating an illusion of relative simplicity. The role of progression in the natural history of cancer points up again the need to look at cancer as a problem in development, or deflection from normal development and function. A basic problem here is that we have a poor grasp of what is involved in normal development, and this in turn is related to a fundamental misapprehension about the nature of living organisms. This shortcoming has been pointed out repeatedly (e.g., 15, 16) and alternative models have been proposed (e.g. 17), but have had little impact on our thinking about development and cancer.

Perhaps this is because it is difficult to find, or even conceive of, a quantitative measure for the degree of organization in cells which are, after all, enormously complex, heterogeneous systems. An approach which has evolved in my laboratory is to measure the metabolic effects of a major cellular cation, magnesium, which regulates a large variety of reactions, and which is also bound to macromolecular and to supramolecular structures in the cell. The affinity of magnesium for these structures according to statistical mechanics is likely to vary with the degree of organization of the structures (17). The affinity of the cells for magnesium, and the dependence of intracellular reactions on its concentration within the cell should serve as an indicator of the metabolically effective state of organization of the cell. Our results along this line thus far (18, 19) lead me to be optimistic about detecting organizational differences between normal and transformed cells. I suspect that progress in this area requires subverting the reductionist, mechanistic assumptions that underlie the current conventions of biological research. Until this happens I fear research in cancer and development will continue to generate a profusion of facts without a comprehensive theory to tie them together in an unforced manner.

Literature Cited

1. Rubin, H. (1980). Is somatic mutation the major mechanism of malignant transformation? *J. Natl. Cancer Instit.* 64, 995-1000.
2. Grobstein, C. (1959). Differentiation of vertebrate cells, in *The Cell,* Academic Press, New York, J. Bracket and A. Mirsky eds.
3. Harris, M. (1964). *Cell Culture and Somatic Variation.* Holt, Rinehart and Winston, New York.
4. Hayflick, L. and Moorhead, P. (1961). The serial cultivation of human diploid cell strains. *Exp. Cell Research,* 25, 585-621.
5. Todaro, G. and Green, H. (1963). Quantitative studies of the growth of mouse embryo cells in culture and their development into established lines. *J. Cell Biol.* 17, 299-313.
6. DeOme, K., Miyamoto, M., Osborn, R., Guzman, R. and Lum, K. (1978). Detection of inapparent nodule - transformed cells in the mammary gland tissue of virgin female BALB/cfC3H mice. *Cancer Res.* 38, 2103-2111.
7. Mintz, B. and Illmensee, K. (1975). Normal genetically mosaic mice produced from malignant teratocarcinoma. *Proc. Natl. Acad. Sci. USA* 72, 3585-3589.
8. Seilern-Aspang, F. and Kratochwil, K. (1965) in *Regeneration in Animals and Related Problems,* ed. V. Kiortsis and H. Trampusch. North-Holland Publishing Co., Amsterdam.
9. Yang, T. and Tobias, C., This Symposium.
10. Mondal, S. and Heidelberger, C. (1970). In vitro malignant transformation by methylcholanthrene of the progeny of single cells derived from c3H mouse prostate. *Proc. Natl. Acad. Sci. USA* 65, 219-229.
11. Parodi, S. and Brambilla, G. (1977). Relationships between mutation and transformation frequencies in mammalian cells treated in vitro with chemical carcinogens. *Mutation Res.* 47, 53-74.

12. Gurdon, J. (1976). Adult frogs derived from the nuclei of single somatic cells. *Develop. Biol.* 4, 256-273.
13. Foulds, L. (1969, 75). *Neoplastic Development*, Vol. I & II, Acad. Press, New York.
14. Cairns, J. (1981). The origins of human cancers. *Nature* 289, 353-357.
15. Elsasser, W. (1961). Quanta and the concept of organismic law. *J. Theoret. Biol.* 1, 27-58.
16. Kacser, H. (1957) in *Strategy of the Genes*, ed. C. Waddington, pp. 191-249.
17. Ling, G. (1962). *A Physical Theory of the Living State.* Blaisdell Publishing Co., New York.
18. Rubin, H. (1981). Growth regulation reverse transformation, and adaptability of 373 cells in decreased Mg^{2+} concentration. *Proc. Natl. Acad. Sci.* USA 78, 328-332.
19. Rubin, H., Vidair, C., and Sanui, H. (1981). *Proc. Natl. Acad. Sci. USA* 78, 2350-2354.

Response of Mice to Varying Times of Ultraviolet Radiation with Implications Toward the Response of Human Beings

Elizabeth L. Scott

Statistical Laboratory
University of California
Berkeley, California

1. Introduction and Summary

We want to study the effects on carcinogenesis that result from changes in administering ultraviolet radiation. The association is with skin cancer which is externally observable, not requiring sacrifice. Therefore, the conclusions obtained are expected to be more reliable than is possible with other types of cancer. Further, the dose information is more complete than with other kinds of cancer, and there are extensive laboratory studies of the effect of ultraviolet radiation on cells, on mice, and on excised human skin. The results will contribute to a better understanding of carcinogenesis and will be applicable in studies estimating the increase in skin cancer that will result from increasing ultraviolet radiation due to depletion by man-made pollution of the absorbing layer of stratospheric ozone.

We first consider the consequences of one change in a fixed scenario of the administration of ultraviolet radiation: intensity, length and pattern of exposures, wavelength spectrum, age at initial exposure, pre-, post-, and continuing exposure to chemicals that are cocarcinogens or coactivators, and so forth. The actual natural scenario is complex; it is not even fixed. There are diurnal and seasonal changes due to the changing position of the sun as well as changes in the atmosphere at all levels -- clouds, pollution and depletion -- that affect the protective absorbtion of ultraviolet radiation. Individuals may react differently to the same ultraviolet radiation due to differences in skin sensitivity, different clothing, different lifestyles. Recent extensive laboratory experiments on mice provide a rich source of the effects of systematic changes in the administration of ultraviolet radiation. We then endeavor to project the conclusions to human beings and to test the implications whenever data are available.

The early experiments of Blum (1959) were designed to provide information on the dose-rate relationships. The ears of a mouse were exposed to ultraviolet radiation, according to a prescribed pattern, producing sarcomas. The rest of the mouse was not exposed, since it was protected by hair in any case.

The recent experiments of Forbes and Urbach (1975-1980) investigated the effects of changing the wavelengths of the ultraviolet radiation as well as other changes. They irradiated a normal, hairless strain of mice, Skh Hairless-1. Each mouse was kept in a separate cage which was exposed to ultraviolet radiation according to the protocol of the experiment. In the latest of these studies, three extensive series of experiments were performed. In the first, a sun-like light source was transmitted through filters of various thickness to simulate the changes in ultraviolet radiation that would occur if the stratospheric ozone were decreased. As discussed below, decreasing the filter thickness increased the incidence of skin cancer on the mice. The second study investigated the effects of altering the length of the daily exposure period while simultaneously altering the thickness of the filter, thus providing a dose-response study which allows the simultaneous study of the effects of changing wavelength. In the third study, the intensity of exposure was varied, as well as the filter thickness. Comparison of the last two studies provides a test of time-dose reciprocity in the selected wavelength range. These studies provide a better understanding of the relationship between changes in the stratospheric ozone layer and the probability that the ultraviolet radiation reaching man from the sun will cause skin cancer.

When the results from experiments on mice are compared with the observations of skin cancer on human beings, we find nothing to contradict any of the projections of the experimental data on mice but certain implications observed on humans are outside of the range of direct projections. In particular, the incidence of malignant melanoma in Norway (Magnus 1981) indicates that simple cumulative dose may be operating over a range of the data but it is not the only factor. High intensity doses may be important. As another particular, we noticed that the slope of the linear relation between the logarithm of the response rate versus ultraviolet flux annual dose is insensitive to age and to sex for human beings, but is larger when individual sites are used rather than the entire body.

2. Results from Experiments with Mice

We will concentrate on some of the features of the interesting experiments of Forbes and Urbach. A concept of importance is the role of the accumulated radiation dose in explaining the incidence of tumors on mice, the build-up of successive tumors, and the growth of tumors. The simple accumulated radiation dose is not sufficient to explain all the experimental results. It is just these deviations from reciprocity that are of special interest in the carry-over of the experimental results from mice to human beings. For example, the extra incidence arising when the dose pattern is broken up into short intervals will be of consequence to human beings. Most people, especially white-collar workers, expose themselves to ultraviolet radiation irregularly and for short time intervals. The results of Forbes (1980) suggest that these individuals will suffer a higher incidence rate of skin cancer than the class of people that work outdoors, thus receiving a rather continuous dose of ultraviolet radiation, even though the total dose accumulated is the same.

Figure 1 shows the increased tumor yield on 24 mice which were exposed for 5 minutes of each of five week-days for 30 weeks in one continuous daily dose (see solid curve), compared to 24 mice which received radiation doses in five daily subdoses of 1 minute each, one hour apart. Thus, the two groups of mice received the same total cumulative dose, but the animals which received the irradiation in the five subdoses tend to have a larger tumor yield and also a larger prevalence of tumors after about

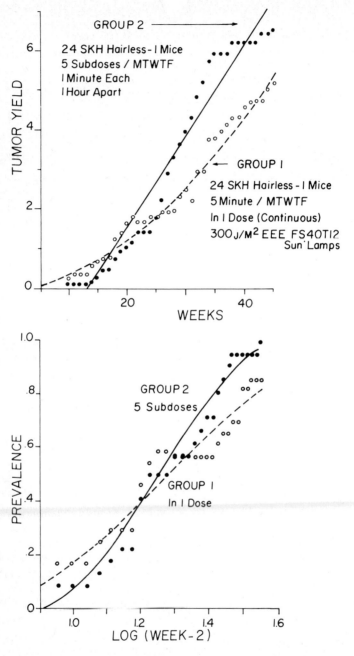

Fig. 1. Increased tumor yield and prevalence after 20 weeks for mice which received same total dose in five subdoses daily. (Adapted from Forbes, Davies, and Urbach (1978)).

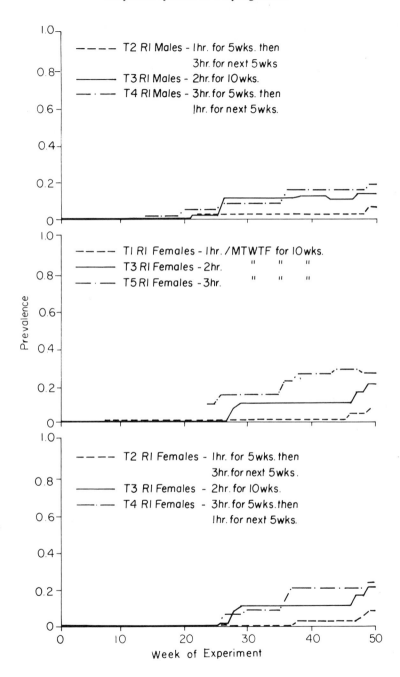

Fig. 2. The effects of dose level and of dose patterns. (Adapted from Forbes, Davies, and Urbach (1979)).

week 20.

The effects of different patterns of doses are contrasted in Figure 2. As shown in the middle panel, one set of 108 animals (labeled T1) received irradiation from a xenon long-arc solar simulator with a 1-mm Schott WG320 glass filter restricting the radiation to the UVB range (approximately 280 to 320 nm) for one hour on the five week-days for 10 weeks. A second set (labeled T3) received two hours per day in the same pattern, and a third set of 108 mice received irradiation for three hours each day. The curves in the middle panel demonstrate an increasing prevalence of tumors according to the increase in dose. In the same series of experiments, a fourth group (labeled T2) received one hour daily for the first 5 weeks, followed by three hours daily for the next 5 weeks, while a fifth group received three hours daily for the first 5 weeks followed by one hour daily for the second 5 weeks. In the upper panel for males and the bottom panel for females we show the resulting prevalence contrasted with the same total dose delivered at a constant rate of two hours per day for 10 weeks. We note that the animals who received the low dose of one hour when younger (followed by the high dose) have the lowest tumor prevalence, well under the curve for a constant dose. After about week 35 following the start of treatment, the animals who received the large dose early have the highest prevalence of tumors. These results reflect the greater sensitivity to carcinogen of the younger animals rather than a special importance of the first half of the treatment, as verified by further experiments starting at 6 weeks of age rather than 16 weeks.

The next two figures contrast the effect of a known chemical cocarcinogen 8-methoxypsoralen applied immediately before each exposure to ultraviolet radiation with that of two fluorescent whitening agents (FWA-I and FWA-III) under test and that of the control vehicle. In both figures and for both measures of response, tumor yield and tumor prevalence, there is a positive interaction between the chemical 8-MOP and the ultraviolet radiation; the effects are seen earlier and they extend higher when compared to the control of irradiation only and when compared to no irradiation (which produced no tumors). On the other hand, the two test chemicals, FWA-I and FWA-III, appear to have responses at the same level or even below the responses from the control vehicle. In Figure 3, the chemicals were applied before each irradiation by treating a 20 cm^2 area in the midback leaving a residue of 0.2 mg of 8-MOP/cm^2 or of 2 mg FWA/cm^2. After 30 to 60 minutes, radiation was started for 10 minutes for a total dose of 90J/m^2 (EEE, erythema effective energy). Both the solution and the radiation were applied daily Monday through Friday for 40 weeks.

In the experiment shown in Figure 4, the animals were bathed by swimming in the solution at a weaker level, leaving a FWA residue of about 1 μg/cm^2 of skin. After 30 to 60 minutes 24 were exposed for 2 hours to a total dose of 300 J/m^2 (EEE) five times each week for 40 weeks, while the remaining 24 were kept as unirradiated controls. Thus, the method of applying the solution, the dose of the chemical and the dose of UV were all different so no clear interpretation of the observed differences is possible. The response levels are different and so are the locations of the tumors: in the first series, most of the tumors developed near the midline of the back but in the second series most of the tumors developed on the animals' sides with very few on the midline. The application of the chemical to a rather small area of the midback appears to influence the location of tumors to the middle line of the back rather than to just the area treated with chemical. On the other hand, when the solution is applied all over except the head, the tumors tend to appear on the sides. With a two hour irradiation, the mice will tend to be sleeping much of the time and thus lying on one side (usually a favorite side) and this may explain the occurrence of tumors on the sides. In the first series, the exposure time was only 10 minutes and was more intense. The animals will not have settled down, which will mean that the dose tended to be applied to the back. Thus, there is confounding between the effects of applying the solution and applying the radiation. In any case, the location of the application does appear to be associated with the location of the tumors, but not precisely.

In their exciting and extensive series of most recent experiments, Forbes, Davies and Urbach (1980) investigate many questions associated with estimating the increases in skin cancer that will accompany decreases in the amount of stratospheric ozone. Two or even three components of the scenario are altered simultaneously, in a systematic way. By installing a series of filters varying from 0.64 to 3.00 mm in thickness, percentage decreases in ozone are simulated, since more, shorter UVB will pass through the thinner filters in a measurable way. In fact, a thinner filter almost corresponds to including an increment of shorter wavelength radiation. In Figure 5 are shown the responses of six groups of 72 Skh Hairless-1 mice each exposed to the same long-arc xenon lamp for 2 hours daily Monday through Friday for 40 weeks. A different filter was used for each group of mice with thickness 0.64, 1.00, 1.3, 2.0 and 3.0 mm respectively. With the thickest filter, the mice receive 119 J/m^2 EEE daily. For each filter thickness, the upper panel of Figure 5 gives the time in weeks since the experiment started until a prescribed proportion - say 0.50 - of the surviving mice have developed at least one tumor. From the lower panel one can read the time to obtain a prescribed tumor yield - say 1.0 tumors per surviving mouse, on the average.

The results are plotted in Figure 6. The time to an average yield of one tumor per survivor and the time to when half the mice have at least one tumor are in good agreement as a function of the filter thickness. When the data are replotted using log time (weeks) versus log daily dose (in EEE), the relation is a straight line with slope -1.6 for median development time (weeks) to first tumor on a mouse, the slope is -1.8 for median development for all tumors observed, and the slope is -1.5 for the time of tumor yield of one tumor per survivor. These results suggest the relation

$$(dose)(time)^p = constant$$

which is the relation found by Blum (1959) for the time to first tumor with p = 2. Forbes' data provide p = 1.6 with a larger experiment. However, the experimental conditions were not the same: Blum irradiated the ears of Swiss mice producing mostly sarcomas, while Forbes irradiates the exposed

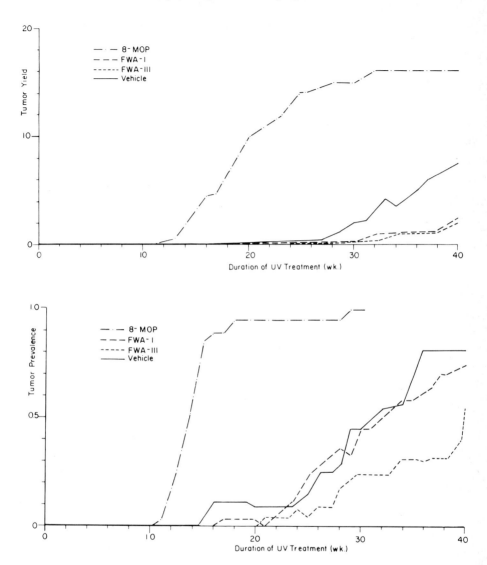

Fig. 3. The effect of pretreatment with chemical applied to small area, followed by UV radiation for 10 minutes daily. (Adapted from Forbes and Urbach (1975a)).

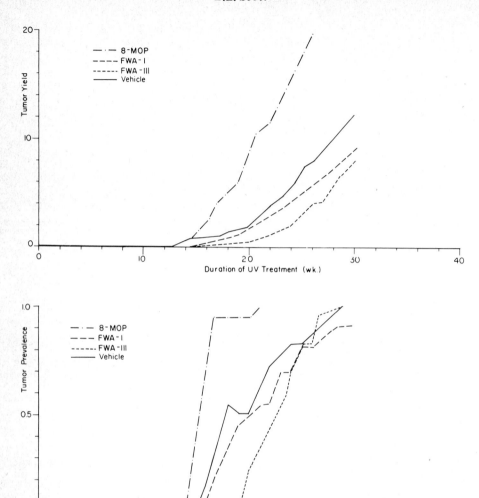

Fig. 4. The effect of pretreatment by bathing in chemical followed by UV irradiation for 2 hours daily. (Adapted from Forbes and Urbach (1975b)).

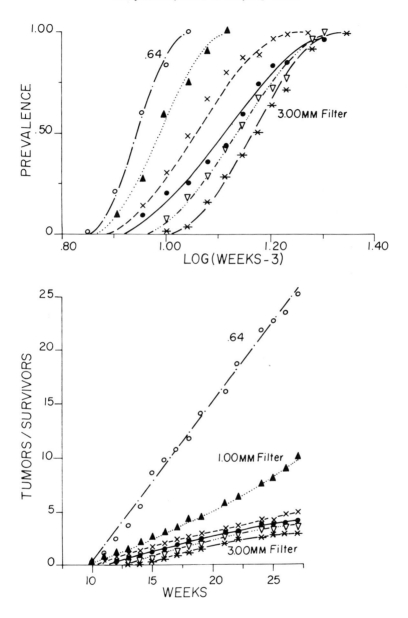

Fig. 5. Response of six groups of mice, each group exposed through different filter thickness for 2 hours daily. (Adapted from Forbes, Davies, and Urbach (1979)).

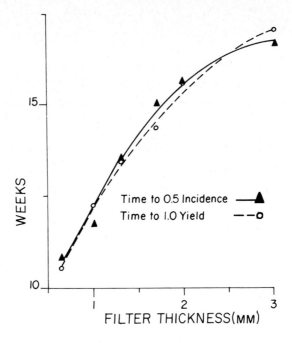

Fig. 6. Time to an average yield of one tumor per survivor and time to when half the mice have at least one tumor are in good agreement. (Adapted from Forbes, Davies, and Urbach (1979)).

parts of the body (usually the side or the back) of hairless mice producing mostly squamous cell carcinoma.

Forbes (1981) demonstrated the differences in response to the same experimental conditions by different strains and different colonies of the same strain. The amount of response at a prescribed time and, correspondingly, the shape of the response curves with time since the start of the experiment are quite different.

In the experiments described up to now, an increase in the dose of ultraviolet radiation administered was achieved by increasing the duration of exposure and/or by decreasing the thickness of the filter. The flux was held constant. However, the dose could have been increased by increasing the flux with exposure period and filter held constant. In the upper part of Figure 7 the prevalence of tumors is shown for mice exposed to a constant flux with a single filter of 1.3 mm thickness, with each group exposed for a different duration, decreasing by about 29% from one group to the next. In the lower panel of Figure 7, the prevalence is shown for groups of mice from the same colony under similar experimental conditions except that now the exposure period is held constant at 2 hours daily for the five days Monday through Friday, the filter is again constant (although shown here at 2.0 mm thickness), and the change in dose is achieved by adjusting the flux decreasing by about 29% from one group to the next. The observed responses have been fitted by logistic curves using logit chi-square in order to estimate the number of weeks to prevalence 0.50. The results suggest that the two methods of dose reduction have the same biological consequences, at least within the limits of these experiments. The authors point out that somewhere outside the experimental limits reciprocity failure does occur, and needs to be taken into account.

3. Results from Observations of Skin Cancer on Human Beings

We now attempt to project the implications of the experimental results from mice to human beings, and then to compare the projections with the available data. Suppose that we project that the logistic shaped response curves carry over as a function of time period of exposure and

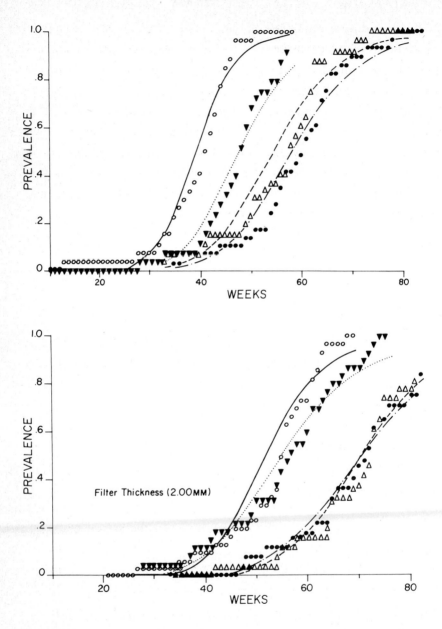

Fig. 7. Prevalence curves for groups administered different doses by adjusting exposure time (upper panel) and by adjusting flux (lower panel). (Adapted from Forbes, Berger, Davies, and Urbach (1980)).

even that the dose multiplied by this time to a power p is constant. For the time period of exposure, consider age as a first approximation. The dose that an individual receives is not now measured. As an approximation, for each locality, we can start by estimating or measuring the instantaneous intensity of ultraviolet radiation per square meter, for example. Such measurements have strong diurnal, annual, and weather-induced variabilities. In the same locality, due to different life-styles, clothing, complexion, and so forth, the dose received under the skin will vary from one person to the next and on different sites of the body of the same person. Thus, even though the mean ultraviolet radiation and the maximum radiation for any location increases toward the equator, the compounding of the many response curves from each locality will diffuse and even bias conclusions drawn from observed rates. The suggestion is to select groups that are as homogeneous as possible on the characteristics implicated by the mice experiments. We now consider the available data and investigate whether the projected relations and differences in relations are present.

Detailed data on malignant melanoma, the more dangerous category of skin cancer, have been reported by Magnus (1981) from the Cancer Registry of Norway. There is an informative chart of the age-specific incidence of malignant melanoma in Norway from 1955 through 1977, done separately by sex and by cohort of birth and for different sites in area units corresponding to one percent of the total skin surface (so that the sites are comparable). When the site considered is face and neck, the log of this incidence shows essentially the same linear relationship with age for both sexes and all cohorts, which indicates that the same sigmoid curve could be used to represent incidence itself as a function of age. However, when the site is trunk or lower limb, which are differentially exposed for the two sexes and for the three cohorts considered (1890-1909, 1910-1929, 1930-1949), the response curves differ, verifying that the incidence rates increase sharply with increased exposure resulting from the sex differences in clothing and the change in attitudes about covering the body swinging through the century from almost complete cover-up even when swimming to deliberate solar exposure virtually unprotected on occasion. For the most recent cohorts, the face-neck area is no longer the most common site. Magnus points out that "it seems justified to assume that at any point of time in life the cumulative dose of sunlight must be larger on the face than on any other site of the body, it can hardly be a simple relationship between the cumulative dose of sunlight and the risk of malignant melanoma."

The shape of the curves show a tendency to level off or even turn down for older ages when log incidence is plotted against age. Magnus suggests that this may be associated with a possible tendency of older persons, especially those who sunburn badly, to avoid acute reactions from sun exposure as a result of experience and lack of social pressure. Since clinical and case-control studies (Sober *et al.* 1979) indicate that serious and repeated sunburn is associated with high risk of malignant melanoma, changes in sunbathing habits may affect the risk of melanoma. The very low rates, non-increasing with age, on the legs of these turn-of-the-century women suggest a deviation from the mice experiment projections if they received the same daily dose of solar radiation on their lower limbs. But they received very small doses, if any, especially the oldest women. Since tanning was not considered to be genteel and clothing was extensive, the legs were well protected.

There are statistical artifacts that may be contributing to a turndown of the observed rates in old age. One is the competing risks of death from other causes. Another is the fact that we are plotting incidence of malignant melanoma for which the median age of being diagnosed is only 40 to 45 years. By definition, a case enters the incidence rates only once, at the year of diagnosis, creating a tendency toward turndown thereafter especially if it is the group of persons with high risk of melanoma who are making the main contribution to the incidence.

We conclude that simple cumulative dose may be operating over a range of the data available for malignant melanoma but it is not the only factor. There is an indication that high intensity doses may be important. Thus, the incidence of malignant melanoma in Norway does not appear to contradict any of the projections of the experimental data on mice, but certain implications are outside of the range of direct projections.

The Health and Nutrition Examination Survey (HANES) data collected by the National Center for Health Statistics (USA) provides detailed dermatological, personal, and health information about 20,749 individuals (of whom 16,262 are white). The data are population proportional samples from 65 stands across the country. Although the sample sizes are small, the HANES data are rich in information about the individual. Many persons show some types of actinic damage to the skin, particularly keratosis, which appears to be a frequent precursor of skin cancer. Therefore, we have augmented the study (Pearl 1979) of the relations between nonmelanoma and the characteristics of the individual by setting up an index of Actinic Damage Severity, which is in maximum likelihood agreement with nonmelanoma incidence. Considering age-specific data, the demographic, dermatological variable that is crucial to the relation with nonmelanoma is the sex of the individual, important are hair color, eye color, ancestry and complexion, which are presumed to represent the vulnerability of the skin. Of secondary importance are acne, senile depigmentation, coarse skin texture, senile purpura, and other selected dermatological disorders. The crucial lifestyle variable is the amount of exposure to sunlight, but also important is the amount of ultraviolet flux of the locality. Also important, but secondary, are exposure to insecticides, immersions, and other possible carcinogens. Using the characteristics listed (except age, sex, and flux, which are considered separately), four categories of risk were established: high, medium, low, and lowest. The possible dependence of predictive variables was not considered when setting up the definitions of risk.

In Figure 8 the average Actinic Damage Severity index is plotted when the entire HANES population has been divided according to sex, age level (young or old), flux level (low or high), and risk group. We see that the lowest ADS occurs for young women, as expected, and that these are much alike with some tendency to increase with higher flux. Older women and young men are roughly similar. Now there is a stronger effect of flux and of risk group, especially for men. The effects are most pronounced for

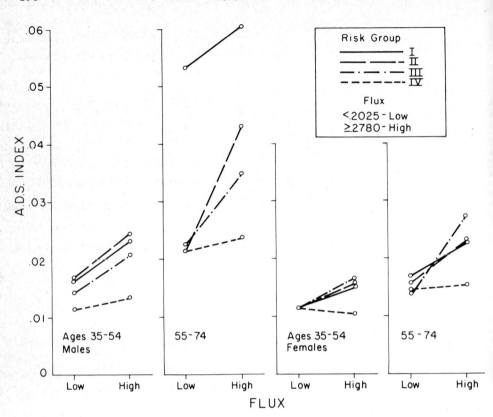

Fig. 8. Actinic Damage Severity Index for different categories of persons in HANES sample: effect of age, sex, flux, and risk group.

older men. The lowest risk group is still well below all others, the low group is higher, especially at high flux, and the medium group rises even more. But the high-risk older males show a very large increase, so that there ADS index is more than twice that of the younger females. This means that the estimated probability of showing nonmelanoma, for a given category, has the same relation. There are not enough cases of melanoma in the HANES data to establish a new ADS index for melanoma. However, there are no contradictions with the ADS established for nonmelanoma. We note that 5 out of the 17 cases of melanoma also had experienced nonmelanoma, all of them older males, with 4 of these from high flux localities.

In order to verify the projections from the mice experiments when the population shows such diverse risk categories, a very large sample would be required, far larger than HANES. We find nothing to negate the projections of the experiments. Again, we find that the observations lie in the lower S-shape of the response curve; most individuals are in categories with relatively low probability of nonmelanoma, but there are abrupt increases in probability when the ultraviolet flux increases and/or the age increases, especially for males. Note that the increases are larger for those groups who already have the bigger probabilities.

Mortality data provide another possibility for verifying the projections from the mice experiments. Through the cooperation of the National Center for Health Statistics, we have information from death certificates for melanoma and nonmelanoma separately. The data include county of residence, age at death, sex, race, and site on body of primary lesion for the years 1968 through 1974. Again using age as a measure of time period of exposure, we can compare the shape of the response curves for mortality with what could be projected from other sorts of response from the mice experiments. Mortality was plotted for successive age intervals separately for males and females and for three intervals of ultraviolet flux of the locality of residence. The age-specific mortality is always largest for the localities with high flux, as would be projected from the mice experiments. The rates for medium flux are intermediate, the rates for the localities with low flux are the smallest. Similar results apply to both males and females, except that the rates for males are much higher. Both sets of curves rise almost linearly for the younger ages and then turn up faster.

The increase in response rate with increasing ultraviolet flux is of special interest. We have empirically investigated various simple functions to approximate the response for the case of mortality, incidence, prevalence, and so forth. In all cases, we find that the logarithm of the response rate versus ultraviolet flux annual dose (say, in photons) provided the best (or essentially the best) fit, no matter which sex, what age interval, what form of skin cancer, etc. is under consideration. Furthermore, the slopes of these loglinear relations are insensitive to age and to sex. Now the slope has the easy interpretation of proportional increase in skin cancer rate that corresponds to unit change in ultraviolet flux.

We noticed that the slope tends to be larger when individual sites on the body are used, rather than the entire body. The slopes obtained by fitting a simple loglinear relation for observed mortality versus flux (Yandell) are shown in the table for the several sites for which there are data from the death certificate. In almost every instance, the slope derived from

Slope of Loglinear Relation Fitting Logarithm of Mortality to Ultraviolet Flux of Locality by Sex and by Site of Lesion

Site on body of lesion	Melanoma		Nonmelanoma	
	Male	Female	Male	Female
Face	3.02	2.40	2.66	1.78
Scalp-neck	2.45	2.54	2.54	2.16
Trunk	3.61	2.77	1.74	1.55
Upper limb	2.36	2.88	2.46	1.97
Lower limb	2.27	1.83	2.44	1.80
Total body	1.42	1.40	2.12	1.34

using the entire body is smaller than the slope obtained by using only those deaths where the primary lesion was at a specified site. The exposure period for individual sites will be less than for the total body. Thus, a different slope could have been predicted from the mice experiments, although the direction of the difference would depend on how one is deviating from a cumulative dose response.

Recent observations of nonmelanoma incidence (Scotto, Fears, and Fraumeni) provide another opportunity to compare results from data on human beings with the projections from experimental mice. We again find that the log of the incidence is linearly related to flux, with nearly the same slope for the two sexes and with the slope for squamous cell carcinoma about double that for basal cell. We again find that the slopes for the individual sites tend to be less than the slope computed for the total body, for both males and females, and for both squamous and basal cell nonmelanoma. Considering the small sample sizes in this special survey sample of the incidence of nonmelanoma, the ratios are roughly maintained with the increases in the upper extremities less well determined but also large. The results for the recent 1977-1978 survey are roughly confirmed by the smaller 1971-1972 survey.

The projections of the mice experiments are not contradicted by the nonmelanoma incidence, although further verification is possible with the data collected but not published. For example, we verify that the flux multiplied by a power of the age at which a prescribed proportion have nonmelanoma is roughly constant, as has been noted by others. It would be interesting to investigate this question for different sites, but this requires access to age-site-sex specific incidence data. On the other hand, response curves for different sites on the mouse would also be of great interest. Since the experimental data of Forbes and the new data by de Gruijl (1982) contain weekly drawings of every experimental mouse, with each tumor numbered and plotted, analyses could be carried out for each site separately. A new experiment in which some sites are exposed less than others (some sites are more protected) would also be of great interest when analyzed for each site separately as compared to analysis for the total animal.

4. Acknowledgements

We are grateful to Dr. P. D. Forbes and Dr. F. Urbach for letting us have the detailed data for one of their experiments, and for interesting and instructive discussions. Many of our investigations are part of our studies under the Panel to Review Statistics on Skin Cancer of the Committee on National Statistics of the National Research Council, and of cooperative studies of an informal Skin Cancer Workshop at the University of California, Berkeley. We are more indebted than we know to Professor Jerzy Neyman, who introduced us to an active study of carcinogenesis and inspired and contributed to further studies.

Some of our studies were performed with the partial support of the National Institute of Environmental Health Sciences (USPHS ESO1299-19 to the University of California, Berkeley and N01-ES-6-2128 to the Committee on National Statistics) and the Environmental Protection Agency (EPA CR8078777-01 to the University of California, Berkeley).

5. References

1. Blum, H. F. *Carcinogenesis by Ultraviolet Light.* Princeton University Press, Princeton, N.J., 1979.

2. Forbes, P. D. Photocarcinogenesis: An overview. *Journal of Investigative Dermatology*, Vol 77: 139-143, 1981.

3. Forbes, P. D., R. E. Davies, D. Berger and F. Urbach. A study on photocarcinogenesis in hairless mice (simulated stratospheric ozone depletion and increased biologically harmful UVR). Final Report, NCI Contract No. NO-1 CP 43271, Center for Photobiology, Temple University 1980.

4. Forbes, P. D., R. E. Davies, and F. Urbach. Aging, environmental influences, and photocarcinogenesis. *Journal of Investigative Dermatology*, Vol 73: 131-174, 1979.

5. Forbes, P. D., R. E. Davies, D. Berger and F. Urbach. Experimental UV photocarcinogenesis: wavelength interactions and time-dose relationships. *National Cancer Institute Monograph* 50: 31-38, 1978.

6. Forbes, P. D. and F. Urbach. Experimental modification of photocarcinogenesis. II. Fluorescent whitening agents and simulated solar UV. *Food Cosmet. Toxicol.* Vol 13: 339-342, 1975a.

7. Forbes, P. D. and F. Urbach. Experimental modicifaction of photocarcinogenesis. III. Simulation of exposure to sunlight and fluorescent whitening agents. *Food Cosmet. Toxicol.* Vol 13: 343-345, 1975b.

8. de Gruijl, F. R. The dose-response relationship for uv-tumorigenesis. Thesis, Utrecht University, 1982.

9. Magnus, Knut. Habits of sun exposure and risk of malignant melanoma: An analysis of incidence rates in Norway 1955-1977 by cohort, sex, age, and primary tumor site. *Cancer,* Vol 48: 2329-2335, 1981.

10. National Center for Health Statistics, United States Department of Health, Education, and Welfare. *Plan and Operation of the Health and Nutrition Survey: United States 1971-1973.* Vital and Health Statistics, Ser. 1, No. 10a. U.S. Govt. Printing Off., Washington, D.C., 1973.

11. Pearl, Dennis. Preliminary analysis of Health and Nutrition Examination Survey. To be published, 1979.

12. Sober, A. J., T. B. Fitzpatrick, and R. Marvell. Solar exposure patterns in patients with cutaneous melanoma -- a case control series. *Clin. Res.* Vol 27: 536A, 1979.

13. Yandell, Brian. Further analysis of mortality: by sex, by site, by race. To be published, 1979.

Viral and Cellular Oncogenes

Hermann Oppermann, M.D.

Department of Microbiology,
University of California,
San Francisco
and Department of Molecular Biology
Genentech, Inc.
San Francisco, California

1. Introduction

RNA tumor viruses have led to the discovery of tumor genes or oncogenes. These oncogenes have proven to be of cellular origin. They represent a set of evolutionary, highly conserved genes, which are usually only moderately active. The physiological function of these genes is regulatory. Certain RNA tumor viruses have incorporated an oncogene into their genome. Evidence accumulates to indicate that the increased activity of such oncogenes is responsible for the malignant state of tumor cells. for once, this can result from infection with an oncogene bearing tumor virus, as viral genes are usually very active. On the other hand, certain mutations may activate the homologous cellular oncogene with the same effect. Thus, hyperactivity of an oncogene seems to be a universal concept of carcinogenesis. The subject is now progressing very rapidly. For other accounts, see (17),(27), (3). Much of our knowledge about the structure and function of genes has come from the study of viruses. Their simple structure, typically a few genes surrounded by a protein shell, was well suited for molecular and genetic analysis. Cancer researchers were attracted because several viruses can cause tumors in animals. Although viruses may play a minor role in human cancer - only the Herpes viruses may be a major cause of it - tumor viruses have been the most rewarding tools of basic cancer research.

2. Retroviruses and Proviruses

Currently great attention is drawn by RNA tumor viruses or retroviruses which we will now discuss. These viruses cause numerous naturally occurring tumors in animals, such as leukemias and sarcomas in cattle, chickens, cats and mice. In addition, they are widespread as permanent residents in the genome of most vertebrate animals.

A retrovirus particle contains its genome in the form of RNA in a shell of core proteins which is enveloped by a lipid membrane and spiked with glycoproteins. The retrovirus genome in its "primordial" form has only three genes; *gag, pol,* and *env,* which encodes coreprotein, polymerase (more specifically reverse transcriptase) and envelope glycoprotein. After infection of a cell the reverse transcriptase produces a DNA copy from the RNA genome of the virus. This viral DNA molecule becomes integrated into the genome of the infected cell and is henceforth treated like cellular genes. In this state it is termed provirus. The infection of germinal cells in this manner has resulted in the permanent association of certain retroviruses with whole animal species (e.g. mice).

The integration of a provirus represents a mutagenic event for the cell. The site of integration may determine the fate of the provirus and, more importantly, of the cell. The cellular genome is a huge reservoir of genes, many of which are dormant while others are always more or less active. Activity of a gene means extensive transcription of messenger RNA (mRNA) by RNA polymerase. The mRNA is translated into the final gene product, a protein, frequently an enzyme. Integration of a provirus may occur at random. Obviously this can be disruptive to the context of cellular gene activity. Moreover, the provirus carries potent signals along with it. On both ends of it, one finds the same long nucleotide stretch. It is termed the "long terminal repeat" (LTR). This nucleotide sequence contains the signals for initiation and termination of RNA transcription. It serves for the ordered transcription of the viral genome.

However, it can also increase the transcription of cellular genes which are flanking the provirus. Recent findings indicate that when certain cellular genes, oncogenes, are stimulated in this way, neoplastic changes occur in the cell.

3. Oncogenes

What is known about oncogenes or cancer genes? The prototype of an oncogene is the sarcoma gene of Rous sarcoma virus (RSV). The history of RSV goes back to 1911 when Peyton Rous showed that a cell free extract prepared from a chicken sarcoma introduced new sarcomas upon injection into other chickens. Decades later the viral nature of this transmissable agent was established. Circa 1970 Steve Martin obtained evidence that the malignant state of Rous sarcoma virus transformed cells was caused by a viral gene. He had isolated mutant viruses which were temperature sensitive with respect to cell transformation. Temperature sensitivity implies a thermolabile protein coded for by a mutated gene. Somewhat later, Peter Duesberg demonstrated that the genome of RSV is larger than that of related nonsarcomagenic viruses. These facts determined the strategy of Stehelin, Varmus and Bishop for their isolation of sarcoma gene DNA.

To understand their procedure we must consider that nucleic acids, DNA and RNA, are long chains of four different nucleotides. The four different nucleotides relate to each other like two couples; each nucleotide likes to hang on to another specific nucleotide. Therefore, a complementary nucleotide sequence or negative copy can be made for any nucleotide chain and will align with it to form the famous "double helix". For the isolation of sarcoma gene DNA, a complementary DNA copy (cDNA) was made using the RNA of Rous sarcoma as template. This was allowed to "base pair" with the genome RNA of a related nonsarcomagenic virus. The *src* cDNA did not find a complement, and thus could be isolated on the basis of single-strandedness. DNA can be labeled radioactively and used as a probe for detection of homologous DNA and RNA. *Src* cDNA was used in this way as a probe for the presence of *src* gene and *src* mRNA in RSV-transformed tumor cells. It was found that cells transformed by RSV contained considerable amounts of *src* mRNA, indicating the active expression of the *src* gene. In contrast, cells which had spontaneously resumed a normal state (reverted) or cured themselves, contained very low levels of *src* mRNA, as expected.

4. Ubiquity of Oncogenes

Very soon the fundamental discovery was made that normal cells not infected by RSV also contained a sarcoma gene and low levels of *src* RNA. This cellular *src* gene (c-*src*) proved to be related to the viral src (v-src), although it was distinguishable from it. The c-*src* gene is present in the cells of all vertebrate animals. Recently it has been found even in the cells of insects. This astonishing degree of gene conservation during evolution of the species indicates a very basic biological function.

An interesting question was whether RSV had spread this gene through the animal kingdom, or whether this virus had adopted a cellular gene. The latter is the case because the *src* gene of RSV is most closely related to the *src* gene of the chicken, which is the permissive host for this virus. Thus RSV had adopted the avian c-*src* gene. Another question is whether the cellular *src* gene itself can cause cancer or whether alterations of it are responsible for the malignant character of the viral *src* gene. Currently the most obvious difference between normal and RSV transformed cells is the level of *src* mRNA. i.e., the level of *src* gene expression. The favored model, therefore, is the Oncogene Hyperexpression model, which says that increase in the level of expression of an oncogene may lead to cell transformation.

This model has been supported by results with many other oncogenic retroviruses. These other viruses differ from RSV in one respect: they have replaced part of the viral genome with a cellular oncogene instead of just attaching it. As a result of this, they are now defective and need "helper" viruses in order to replicate. This created some difficulty during the investigation of the defective tumor viruses. Despite this, more than a dozen different retroviruses were found bearing oncogenes distinct from *src.* These viruses were isolated from chickens, mice, cats, etc., and produce sarcomas, different forms of leukemias, and some carcinomas. From this, it appears that different oncogenes have different target tissues, i.e., some oncogenes will only cause sarcomas in connective tissues, others only cancer of the blood cells, and others cancers in certain organs. This target specificity of oncogenes is also observed after infection of cultured tissues. The *src* gene of RSV leads to rapid transformation of fibroblasts, but does not seem to affect epithelial cells. The *myb* gene of myeloblastosis virus malignant transformation of cultured myeloblasts but not of fibroblasts.

As more oncogenes are being discovered, we want to know how many there are altogether. Perhaps a cautious estimate could be made, based on how often the same oncogene was discovered in retroviruses of different species. As of now, only one oncogene has been discovered repeatedly in viruses of different species; the feline sarcoma gene is also found in two different chicken sarcoma viruses. The gene is called *fes* and *fps*, respectively. Another consideration is that the majority of known oncogenes appear to be sarcoma genes. This is due in part to the method of their isolation, namely, as viruses which cause morphological transformation in fibroblasts. Fibroblasts are the favored type of tissue culture cells, because they are easy to culture. However, carcinomas of various organs are the most frequent forms of human cancer. Nevertheless, we still have to discover all those carcinoma-specific oncogenes.

In a way, cancer research was fortunate to have found the defective oncogenic viruses, because they proved very resourceful. There are other oncogenic retroviruses which manage to cause malignancy without carrying an oncogene around. Only very recently has it been found that these viruses succeed in this by positioning themselves and their LTR near one of the cellular oncogenes. The LTR then cause hyperactive transcription of such a cellular oncogene, creating malignant growth.

5. Mechanism of malignant transformation

So far we have not discussed the final mechanism by which the *src* gene or other oncogenes cause the malignant cell transformation. A gene represents the blueprint for the synthesis of its gene product. Not all the oncogene gene products have been found yet, but a good deal is known about the *src* gene product. It was discovered by Brugge and Erickson using reaction with specific antisera. These antisera were obtained from young rabbits which at birth were injected with a high dose of RSV and which later developed sarcomas. The *src* protein is a protein kinase, an enzyme that modifies other proteins by the addition of phosphate. This type of modification is known to have regulatory effects. The discovery of this function came as a surprise: Addition of a suitable phosphate donor to an immune complex containing the *src* protein resulted in phosphate transfer to the antibody. The site of phosphorylation on the antibody, the amino acid tyrosine, was unusual. Phosphorylation of antibody is not the natural function of the *src* protein. However, phosphorylation of tyrosine is rare enough that, in the search for the substrate of *src*, it narrowed the choice of natural targets of the *src* protein. These seem to be molecules related to cell-to-cell contact and cell anchorage. Both of these functions are severely altered in tumor cells.

Similar functions were found for some of the other oncogene proteins, but much remains to be learned. Shared by many oncogenes also is the intracellular localization, which could be either in the cell nucleus, in an organelle, in the cytoplasm, or inside or outside the cell membrane. Many oncogene proteins have been found on the inside of the cell membrane. This fact also hints at some common mechanisms of action.

What then is the physiological role of the cellular oncogenes? Built-in self destruction? As the phosphorylation activity of the *src* protein indicates, oncogenes have a regulatory function. It must be a rather vital function, because the oncogenes are so extremely well conserved during evolution. The localization of oncogene proteins at the cell membrane and at points of cell-to-cell contact hints at functions of communication. A role for oncogenes during the development of multicellular organisms is suspected. Trouble in communications systems can lead to disaster.

6. Prospects

New prospects have been created by the rapid development of recombinant DNA technology, which has also accelerated the investigation of oncogenes. The most beneficial result has been the isolation of the cellular oncogenes and the determination of their nucleotide sequence. From the nucleotide sequence, the primary and secondary protein structure can be deduced. Furthermore, in cases where natural antisera directed against the respective oncogene have been unavailable, these can now be raised. To this end, bacteria are employed to translate the oncogene into its protein product with high efficiency. It is hoped that the antisera and cDNA probes will allow the correlation of oncogenes with human tumors. If so, they may also provide a rapid means of diagnosis and screening.

7. References

1. Bishop, J. Michael. The Molecular Biology of RNA Tumor Viruses: A Physician's Guide. *New England Journal of Medicine*, Vol. 303, No. 12, p. 675, September 1980.

2. Bishop, J. Michael. Enemies Within: The Genesis of Retrovirus Oncogenes. *Cell*, 303, p. 675, December 1980.

3. Bishop, J. Michael. Oncogenes. *Scientific American*, 246, p. 80, March 1982.

Metastatic and Systemic Factors in Neoplastic Progression

Robert Bartoszyński, 1, 2, 3)

Barry W. Brown, 2, 3)

James R. Thompson, 2, 3)

1) Visiting Mathematician from Institute of Mathematics, Polish Academy of Sciences, 00-950 Warsaw, Poland

2) Department of Biomathematics, U. T. M. D. Anderson Hospital, Houston, Texas 77030

3) Department of Mathematical Sciences, Rice University, Houston, Texas 77001

ABSTRACT

A stochastic model of neoplastic progression is developed in which there are two mechanisms for the spread of a tumor. The first represents the traditional metastatic mechanism and posits that the probability of a new tumor occurrence is proportional to the total tumor burden. The second mechanism we term systemic, and it contributes a small but constant probability of new tumor occurrence.

The model yields an excellent fit to a set of breast cancer data, and the same data cannot be adequately fit by the same model with the systemic mechanism disabled. We conclude that some process in addition to the traditional metastatic mechanism must be operative.

1. Introduction

A traditional view [5] of neoplastic progression is that an exponentially growing primary tumor disseminates potential metastases at a rate proportional to its size. Previous investigation [2] showed that the hazard rate of discovery of new tumors after removal of the primary tended to be flat or decreasing in many cases. This fact is inconsistent with the above view even if allowance is made for the time required for the metastasis to grow to detectable size.

Because of this inconsistency we suggest a model in which the metastatic mechanism is supplemented by a systemic mechanism which yields a low but constant rate of formation of new tumors independent of the status of the primary tumor. We shall call tumors originating from the latter mechanism *quasimetastases*. The blanket term for both metastases and quasimetastases will be simply *secondary tumors*.

The general type of data which we consider is as follows. The zero time point for each patient is the time of treatment of the primary tumor. The total time of observation of the patient, S, is known, as is whether or not the patient displayed a secondary tumor and, if so, the time S' of detection of the secondary tumor. A commonly occurring case is that only the time to the first new tumor is recorded so that $S = S'$ for those patients with a secondary tumor. Extension of the model to consider more than one secondary tumor is straightforward but is not presented because such data sets are not common and the computational effort in fitting such data increases exponentially with the number of secondary tumors considered.

We assume that when a secondary tumor is observed, it is not known whether it is a metastasis or quasimetastasis, although the cell type originating the tumor is sometimes determinable. Cells from the originating primary tumor could cause systemic behavior through long quiescence terminated by a randomly occuring perturbation.

Our main question may now be formulated as follows: are the data on temporal characteristics of the waiting times S' for secondary tumors compatible with the hypothesis that only metastatic (but not systemic) component operates in tumor origination? To answer this question we build a model, presented in subsequent sections, and use a sample of patients to estimate the relevant parameters.

To reasonably approximate the assumption that the size of the primary tumor is the factor determining the probability of detection, we choose the patients whose primary tumor was in the breast. In order to reasonably satisfy other assumptions of the model, concerning the growth of possible metastatic and quasimetastatic tumors, we took into the sample only those patients whose primary tumor was classified, at the time of detection, as "category 1" (least serious). For such patients the primary tumor was removed, but no mastectomy was performed, lymph nodes were not affected, and no chemo- or radiotherapy was applied. In short, at the time of removal of the primary, no actions were taken which would affect the growth of any secondary tumors existing at that time.

2. The Model

Hypothesis 1. *For any patient, each tumor originates from a single cell, and grows at a rate α. The latter varies between patients according to the distribution $G(u) = P(\alpha \leq u)$.*

Hypothesis 2. *The probability of systemic occurrence of a tumor in $(t, t+\Delta t)$ equals $\lambda \Delta t + o(\Delta t)$, independent of the prior history of the patient.*

To formulate the remaining hypotheses, let $Y_0(t)$, $Y_1(t)$, $\cdots$, denote the sizes of the primary and secondary tumors at t, the subscript representing the order in which they originate.

Hypothesis 3. *The probability that the primary tumor will be detected and removed in $(t, t+\Delta t)$ is $bY_0(t) \Delta t + o(\Delta t)$, and until the removal of the primary, the probability of a metastasis in $(t, t+\Delta t)$ is $aY_0(t) \Delta t + o(\Delta t)$.*

For the remaining hypotheses, consider first the patients with no discovery of secondary tumors in the time of observation, S, and put $m_1(t) = Y_1(t) + Y_2(t) + \cdots$.

Hypothesis 4. *After removal of the primary, the probability of a metastasis in $(t, t+\Delta t)$ equals $am_1(t)\Delta t + o(\Delta t)$, while the probability of detection of a tumor in $(t, t+\Delta t)$ is $bm_1(t)\Delta t + o(\Delta t)$.*

Consider now patients who do display a secondary tumor, and let $m_2(t) = Y_2(t) + Y_3(t) + \cdots$.

Hypothesis 5. *After removal of the primary and before removal of $Y_1(t)$, the probability of detection of a tumor in $(t, t+\Delta t)$ equals $bY_1(t)\Delta t + o(\Delta t)$, while the probability of a metastasis is $aY_1(t)\Delta t + o(\Delta t)$.*

Hypothesis 6. *After removal of $Y_1(t)$, the probability of a metastasis in $(t, t+\Delta t)$ is $am_2(t)\Delta t + o(\Delta t)$, while the probability of detection of a tumor is $bm_2(t)\Delta t + o(\Delta t)$.*

Let us denote by T_0 the (unobservable) time which elapses between the moment when the primary tumor originates and when it is detected and removed (at $t=0$). Similarly, T_1 and T_2 are the times (counted from $t=0$) until detection and removal of the first and second of the subsequent tumors. To write down the likelihood function of the sample of patients, we need the probabilities $P(T_1>S)$ for patients with no detected secondary tumor and probabilities $P(T_1 = S', T_2 > S)$ for patients with a secondary tumor detected at time S'.

The parameters of the model are: λ = rate of spontaneous tumor occurrence, a = rate of metastatic progression, and b = detection rate. The distribution function G governing the between-patient tumor growth rate is assumed given.

Constrained by the difficulty of solving equations which result from the model, we introduce the following auxiliary hypotheses.

We refer to the period prior to detection of the primary as phase 0. Phase 1 is the period from detection of the primary to S', the first time of detection of a secondary tumor. For those without a secondary tumor, phase 1 is the time of observation, S. Phase 2 is the time, if any, between S' and S.

Hypothesis 7. *For patients who do not display a secondary tumor, growth of the primary tumor, and of all tumors in phase 1, is deterministically exponential; the growth of all other tumors is treated as a pure birth process.*

Hypothesis 8. *For patients who display a secondary tumor, the growth of the following tumors is treated as deterministic: in phase 0 - tumors $Y_0(t)$ and $Y_1(t)$; in phase 1 - tumor $Y_1(t)$ and all tumors which originated in phase 0; in phase 2 - all tumors. The growth of remaining tumors in phases 0 and 1 is treated as a pure birth process.*

3. The Theoretical Analysis

Let us denote now

$$H(s;t,z) = \exp\left\{\frac{az}{\alpha} e^{\alpha t} (e^s - 1) \log[1 + (e^{-\alpha t} - 1) e^{-s}]\right.$$
$$\left. + \frac{\lambda}{\alpha} s - \frac{\lambda}{\alpha} \log[1 + e^{\alpha t}(e^s - 1)]\right\}, \quad (1)$$

and

$$p(t;z) = bze^{\alpha t} \exp[-\frac{bz}{\alpha}(e^{\alpha t} - 1)]. \quad (2)$$

Suppose that the primary tumor originated at time $-\tau$, and remained undetected until time $t=0$. Let X be the total mass of all tumors excluding the primary at time $t=0$. We have then

Proposition 1. *The Laplace transform of X is given by*

$$Ee^{-sX} = H(s;\tau,1). \quad (3)$$

Proof. Clearly, $X = X_1 + X_2$, where X_1 and X_2 are contributions to X from the metastases and quasi-metastases.

The Laplace transform of X_1 can be obtained from formula (10.61) of Bailey [1]. In the present notations, this formula yields

$$Ee^{-sX_1} = \exp\left\{\frac{a}{\alpha} e^{\alpha \tau}(e^s - 1) \log[1 + (e^{-\alpha \tau} - 1) e^{-s}]\right\}. \quad (4)$$

To get the distribution of X_2 let

$$K(s,\tau) = \log E e^{sX_2}. \tag{5}$$

It is not difficult to show that $K(s,\tau)$ must satisfy

$$\frac{\partial K}{\partial \tau} - \alpha(e^s - 1)\frac{\partial K}{\partial s} = \lambda(e^s - 1) \tag{6}$$

with $K(s,0) = 1$.

The solution of (6) is easily found to be

$$K(s,\tau) = -\frac{\lambda}{\alpha}s - \frac{\lambda}{\alpha}\log[1 - e^{\alpha\tau}(1-e^{-s})]. \tag{7}$$

Taking exponentials and changing s to $-s$ we obtain from (7) the Laplace transform of X_2. Since X_1 and X_2 are independent, multiplying the last result by (4) we prove Proposition 1.

Proposition 2. *The density of the random variable T_0 is equal to $p(t;1)$.*

Proof. By Hypotheses 1, 3 and 7, the detection intensity for the primary tumor is $be^{\alpha t}$. Thus

$$P\{T_0 > \tau\} = \exp\{-b\int_0^\tau e^{\alpha t} dt\} = \exp\{-\frac{b}{\alpha}(e^{\alpha\tau}-1)\}. \tag{8}$$

Differentiating we obtain Proposition 2.

Finally, for patients who do not display a secondary tumor, we have Proposition 3.

$$P(T_1 > S \mid X = x) = e^{-xv(S) + w(S)} \tag{9}$$

where

$$w(y) = \lambda\left[\int_0^y e^{-v(u)} du - y\right] \tag{10}$$

and $v(u)$ is determined from

$$u = \int_0^v (a + b + \alpha s - ae^{-s})^{-1} ds. \tag{11}$$

Proof. Denote

$$P\{T_1 \geq t \mid X=x\} = U(x,t). \tag{12}$$

Until the first occurrence of a new tumor the total mass $m(t)$ grows exponentially with $m(t) = xe^{\alpha t}$. This yields the density of time ξ of the occurrence of the first tumor after 0 to be

$$(\lambda + ae^{\alpha y}) \exp\left[-\lambda y - \frac{ax}{\alpha}(e^{\alpha y}-1)\right]. \tag{13}$$

Take now any s with $0 \leq s \leq t$. Conditioning with respect to $\xi > s$ and $\xi = y \leq s$ we get

$$U(x,t) = \exp\left[-\lambda s - \frac{ax}{\alpha}(e^{\alpha s}-1)\right]$$

$$\cdot \exp\left[-\frac{bx}{\alpha}(e^{\alpha s}-1)\right] U(xe^{\alpha s}, t-s) +$$

$$+ \int_0^s (\lambda + axe^{\alpha y}) \exp\left[-\lambda y - \frac{ax}{\alpha}(e^{\alpha y}-1)\right]$$

$$\cdot \exp\left[-\frac{bx}{\alpha}(e^{\alpha y}-1)\right] U(xe^{\alpha y}+1, t-y)\, dy. \tag{14}$$

Taking $s = \Delta t$, the Taylor expansion yields

$$\frac{\partial U(x,t)}{\partial t} = \alpha x \frac{\partial U(x,t)}{\partial x} - [\lambda + (a+b)x] U(x,t)$$

$$+ (\lambda + ax) U(x+1, t). \tag{15}$$

The initial condition is here $U(x,0) = 1$ for all $x \geq 0$.

Looking for a solution of the form $U(x,t) = \exp\{-xv(t) + w(t)\}$ we find easily the equations for $v(t)$ and $w(t)$ and check that (10) and (11) are the desired solutions.

From Propositions 1 - 3 we obtain

Proposition 4. *For patients who develop metastases, we have*

$$P(T_1 > S) = P(\text{no secondary tumor in } (0,S)) =$$

$$\int_0^\infty \int_0^\infty e^{w(S)} \, p(t;1) \, H(v(s); t,1) \, dt \, dG(\alpha). \tag{16}$$

In a similar way we obtain

Proposition 5. *For patients who do display a secondary tumor we have*

$$P(T_1 = S', T_2 > S) =$$

$$\int_0^\infty \int_0^\infty \int_0^t e^{w(S-S')} \, p(t;1) \, p(S'; e^{\alpha u}) \, (\lambda + ae^{\alpha(t-u)})$$

$$\exp\left[-\lambda(t-u) - \frac{a}{\alpha}(e^{\alpha(t-u)} - 1)\right] H(v(S-S'); S', e^{\alpha u})$$

$$H(v(S-S') \, e^{\alpha S'}; u, e^{\alpha(t-u)}) \, du \, dt \, dG(\alpha)$$

$$+ \int_0^\infty \int_0^\infty \int_0^{S'} e^{w(S-S')} \, p(t;1) \, \exp\left[-\lambda t - \frac{a}{\alpha}(e^{\alpha t}-1)\right] \lambda e^{-\lambda u}$$

$$\cdot p(S'-u;1) \, H(v(S-S'); S'-u, 1) \, du \, dt \, dG(\alpha). \tag{17}$$

4. Results

Data on time in months to first discovery of a secondary tumor on 116 women presenting with localized breast disease were collected by Director Koszarowski, Professor Gadomska and mgr. Kupść at the Curie-Sklodowska Cancer Institute in Warsaw. The distribution of α was taken as concentrated at a single point and maximum likelihood estimation of the parameters from this data was obtained using STEPIT [3]. Estimated parameter values were $a = .17 \times 10^{-9}$, $b = .23 \times 10^{-8}$, $\alpha = .31$ and $\lambda = 0.0030$. Figure 1 presents the Kaplan-Meier estimates of the proportion free of discovered secondary tumors and the proportion from the model with the parameter values given. The agreement of the model with the data appears excellent.

Some consequences of the parameter values may be immediately inferred. For example, tumor doubling time is 2.2 months. The median time from primary origination to detection is 59.2 months and at this time

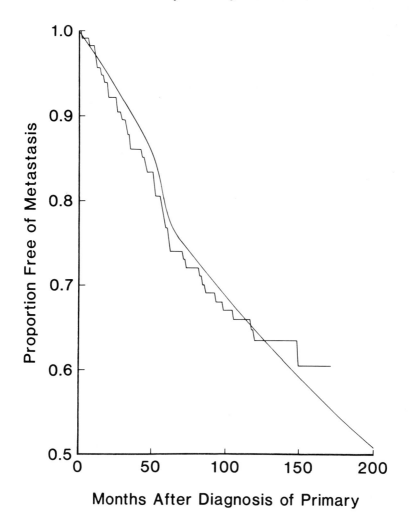

Figure 1. Kaplan-Meier estimate of time to metastasis and the fit obtained from the model for breast cancer data.

the tumor consists of 9.3×10^7 cells. The mean time to quasimetastasis due to the systemic process alone is 27.7 years. The probability of metastasis prior to detection of the primary is 0.069.

An attempt was made to fit the same model, without the systemic mechanism, to the data. The attempt failed. The fitting procedure tried to drive a and α to 0 and the likelihoods were much smaller than in the full model.

In Table 1 below, we examine the relative significance of the metastatic and systemic processes. We note that for all time values examined, the cumulative risk of secondary tumor formation from the systemic process is greater than that from the metastatic process.

Table 1

Probability of One or More Metastases
From Two Mechanisms
Before Various Times from Primary Origination

Time (Years)	Metastatic Mechanism	Systemic Mechanism
1	2.26×10^{-8}	.0354
2	9.34×10^{-7}	.0695
3	3.85×10^{-5}	.102
4	1.57×10^{-3}	.134
5	.0423	.165
6	.0688	.194
10	.0688	.302

5. Discussion

This model is based on simplification as are all models. Probably the most important simplification is the assumption of constancy of the parameters of the model: a, the rate of metastatic progression; b, the detection rate; α, the growth rate (as employed in fitting the data); and λ, the rate of systemic progression. This assumption presupposes that the inter-person variation is small.

There are assumptions introduced purely for mathematical tractability. Those specified in Hypotheses 7 and 8 assert the character of the growth of the tumor and seem to be harmless enough: when the tumor reaches some threshold size, e.g., 1000 cells, it matters little whether one treats its growth as deterministic or not.

For reasons of tractability Hypotheses 3 and 4 were introduced, according to which the metastases may occur only from the primary tumor in Phase 0, while in Phase 1, probability of detection depends on the total tumor mass. One can presume that in exponentially growing tumors, the size of one will dominate the others, determining the metastasis and detection rates.

The full model fits the data set quite well, whereas the model with the systemic process disabled could not achieve an acceptable fit. We consider this evidence that some mechanism must be operating other than the traditional metastatic process whose intensity is proportional to the size of the primary tumor.

6. Acknowledgements

The authors gratefully acknowledge the expert programming of Neely Atkinson. This work was supported in part by Grant CA11430 from the National Cancer Institute and grant DAAG29-78-G-0187 from the U. S. Army Research Office. Dr. Bartoszyński was partially supported by a Yamagiwa-Yoshida Memorial International Cancer Study Grant.

7. References

[1] Bailey, N. T. J. *The Elements of Stochastic Processes with Applications to the Natural Sciences.* New York. 1967. Wiley.

[2] Bartoszyński, R., Brown, B. W., McBride, C. M. and Thompson, J. R. (1981) "Some non-parametric techniques for estimating the intensity function of a cancer-related nonstationary Poisson process". *Annals Stat.* Vol. 9, No. 5, pp. 1050-1060.

[3] Chandler, J. P. (1975) **STEPIT**. Distributed by Quantum Chemistry

Exchange, University of Indiana, Bloomington, Indiana.

[4] Le Cam, L. "On some mathematical models of tumor growth and metastases". (1981). Chapter in the present volume.

[5] Liotta, L. A., Saidel, G., Kleinerman, J., and DeLisi, C. (1977) in *Cancer Invasion and Metastasis: Biologic Mechanisms and Therapy.* ed. Day, S. B. (Raven, New York) pp. 485-491.

On Some Mathematical Models of Tumor Growth and Metastasis

L. Le Cam

University of California, Berkeley

1. Introduction

A study of the temporal patterns by which tumors shed metastasis producing cells and grow is of interest by itself. It is also of importance for prognosis and for patient management. There is an extensive literature on the subject, much of it using terms such as "exponential growth" and referring to "doubling times". (That is the time it takes for a tumor to double its volume) A simple stochastic model based on the same general idea uses the classical birth and death processes. The present author's own, very limited, experience did not predispose him to believe that any such simple model could possibly mimic reality in detail. There is however a possibility that it could reproduce some of the gross features of the situation. A recent study by Bartoszyński and others of the times of discovery of further tumors after breast surgery claims that a birth and death model does reproduce the observations if one adds to the metastatic process a supplement in the form of spontaneous new primaries. In the present paper we discuss a similar model, intended mostly for application to osteogenic sarcoma. The main conclusion is that the human population must be considered wildly heterogeneous. This heterogeneity is not limited to what can be introduced in a birth and death model by letting each patient follow his own arbitrary time scale.

Some of the medical relevance of studies on tumor growth is mentioned in Section 2 below. This same section recounts anecdotal evidence indicating the complexity of the situation. Section 3 elaborates a simple birth and death model for the case of a single individual. Section 4 indicates why such a model fails to cope with very gross observations on osteogenic sarcoma and why the heterogeneity in the patient population must extend beyond differences in time scales. The conclusion will not surprise medically oriented observers. However it does not seem to be well known in statistical circles.

2. Relevance and Anecdotes

The medical literature on the kinetics of tumor growth is extensive. A fairly recent account on the subject can be found in the book by G. G. Steel, [8]. A rapid perusal of one journal, *Cancer*, for breast carcinoma only, yielded 7 articles on the subject. Some of the papers, for instance [5] show a definite correlation between the doubling times of the tumor and the length of survival of the patient. Another study [7] reaches the conclusion that tumor growth is primarily exponential with doubling times varying from patient to patient according to a lognormal distribution. It uses the survival of the patients beyond that predicted from his doubling time as a measure of effectiveness of palliative therapy. Joseph *et. al.* in [4] use doubling times of pulmonary metastasis for prognostic purposes, recommending surgical resection if the doubling times exceed 40 days whether the metastasis are isolated or multiple. They indicate that, for doubling times inferior to 20 days, surgical intervention may subject the patient to unnecessary and undesirable stress without prolonging life materially. The kinetics of tumor growth have also been involved in tentative explanations of differences according to centers in the effects of total lung irradiation, since 2000 rads is expected to be able to eradicate only very small tumor masses. (More than 2000 rads would induce fibrosis.)

The present author has had personal experience with requesting that pulmonary metastasis be surgically resected in the case of two separate patients. In one case, with doubling time of about five or six days, a surgeon temporized and then excused himself saying that "if it grows that fast, it should not be removed." Another surgeon was persuaded to proceed. The patient is live, free of disease, eight years after the surgery. In the second case, with doubling time approximately 20 days, it took four months to find a surgeon willing to operate. One surgeon said "Mr. Le Cam, you know as well as I do that he will die. Why torture him?" The patient did die.

It is an accepted fact that tumors grow "primarily exponentially" but also in a irregular manner. See [8] page 17 for an illustration. The rates of growth vary not only from patient to patient but also for different metastases from the same tumor, even if located close to each other in the same lung. To illustrate some of the possibilities here are two anecdotes taken from my own very limited experience. Patient X had a leg removed at diagnostic of osteogenic sarcoma of the proximal femur. Six months later two nodules were seen in the lung. One month later, they could not be detected on repeat radiographies. Ten months afterwards they reappeared in the same position. The patient died a year later. Patient Y presented with an osteogenic sarcoma of the proximal tibia. It was treated by high dose irradiation. Twenty-eight months later the tumor had crossed over the knee joint and the patient had three lung metastases. This patient underwent a series of treatments, including immunotherapy, chemotherapy, radiation and multiple thoracotomies. During the chemotherapy and radiation treatments some metastases decreased in size, some grew and new metastases occurred. The treatments were discontinued when they were felt to induce life threatening immunodeficiency (WBC < 400). Since then, that is for six years, the patient has no treatment and no noticeable change in the number or size of the metastases. Obviously, such behavior is hardly compatible with the usual birth and death process descriptions. Other somewhat unusual observations may be. For instance in a series of 46 consecutive patients thoracotomized at the Mayo Clinic one finds a patient who had a lung metastasis diagnosed and removed 10 years after treatment of the primary. (The median time to appearance is about 6 months.) For another patient in the same series the primary could not be found, even at autopsy.

Recently R. Bartoszyński, B. W. Brown and J. R. Thompson [1], [2] have used a sophisticated statistical technique to analyze data on breast-cancer from the Curie-Sklodowska Cancer Institute in Warsaw. These authors conclude that the data is incompatible with a birth and death process description unless one allows for a sizable rate of occurrence of new primaries. In this author's view the conclusion is premature. The model used does not allow for sufficient variability of growth rates from person to person. (The reported doubling times for breast cancer range from 4 days to 950.) In the case of breast cancer there may be a possibility that a new primary in the breast may be confused with a metastasis. This is definitely not the case for pulmonary metastases of osteosarcoma. Data of this kind could be used to check the performance of the method described in [2].

However, as we shall explain below, other forms of heterogeneity must be taken into consideration.

3. The Birth and Death Linear Model

In the present section we elaborate some formulas relative to a birth and death process intended to represent what may happen in *one* individual patient. Discussion of *groups* of patients will be given later in Section 4.

The model most often used to describe tumor growth is a simple linear birth and death model according to the following assumptions.

(A1). *The cells act and divide independently of each other. In an interval $(t, t+h]$ a cell can either do nothing, divide with probability $\lambda h + o(h)$, or die with probability $\mu h + o(h)$. We assume $\lambda > \mu$.*

(A2). *The number of live cells in the tumor is one at time zero. It is $N(t)$ at time t, and $N(t)$ is a Markov process.*

(A3). *The probability that a tumor be discovered in $(t, t+h]$ is $\gamma_2 N(t) h + o(h)$.*

(A4). *The probability that a metastasis originates during $(t, t+h]$ is $\gamma_1 N(t) h + o(h)$.*

These are essentially the assumptions of [2]. The authors consider not only metastases originating from the primary tumor but further metastases originating from the first ones and so forth *ad infinitum*. We shall concern ourselves only with the metastases originating from the primary.

Note that (A4) involves the probability of a metastasis originating in $(t, t+h]$. We shall assume that it grows according to a birth and death process. Thus, it may happen that the process dies out and that the metastasis will never be observed.

(A5). *The metastases grow independently of each other and of the primary according to a birth and death process with coefficients* λ_1 *and* μ_1 *(as in (A1), (A2))*.

According to these assumptions, the probability that either a birth or a death will occur in the primary during $(t, t+h]$ is $(\lambda+\mu) N(t) h + o(h)$. Hence the appellation "linear". This assumption is not realistic for very large tumors because of focal necrosis and other phenomena. However these may be ignored for tumors of ordinary clinically detectable size. The assumptions also ignore a host of other phenomena, such as 1) the induction of immune tolerance by large tumors, 2) the secretion of angiogenetic factors insuring good blood supply to the tumor, 3) the influence of the tumor shape on the probabilities of detection or release of metastatic cells, 4) many others which cannot be listed here. Since our purpose is partly to discuss the difficulties of possible applications to *groups* of patients, we shall proceed even though the model is obviously simplistic.

For simplicity, let us say that an event occurs at t if the primary is discovered at t or if a metastasis originates at t. Then, under (A1) to (A5) and conditionally given the entire process $\vec{N} = \{N(t): t \geq 0\}$, the probability that no event occurs before t is $\exp\{-(\gamma_1+\gamma_2) \int_0^t N(x)\, dx\}$. One can readily obtain an expression for the function

$$Q(u, t) = E u^{N(t)} \exp\{-(\gamma_1+\gamma_2) \int_0^t N(x)\, dx\}. \tag{1}$$

Indeed, let $0 \leq u_1 \leq u_2$ be the solutions of the equation $\lambda u^2 - (\lambda+\mu+\gamma_1+\gamma_2) u + \mu = 0$. Let

$$\beta = \lambda(u_2 - u_1) = \{(\lambda-\mu)^2 + 2\gamma(\lambda+\mu) + \gamma^2\}^{1/2},$$

with $\gamma = \gamma_1+\gamma_2$. Then $0 \leq u_1 \leq 1 \leq u_2$ and

$$Q(u, t) = u_1 + \frac{(u_2-u_1)(u-u_1)}{(u_2-u)\exp\{\beta t\} + (u-u_1)}. \tag{2}$$

These formulas are easily derived. They can be found for instance in [6].

The probability that no event occurs before t is then $Q(1, t)$ so that

$$Q(1, t) = u_1 + \frac{(u_2-u_1)(1-u_1)}{(u_2-1)\exp\{\beta t\} + (1-u_1)}. \tag{3}$$

The probability that no event occurs in $(0, \infty)$ is u_1. The conditional probability that no event occurs before t given that an event occurs in $(0, \infty)$ is $(u_2-u_1)[(u_2-1)\exp\{\beta t\} + 1 - u_1]^{-1}$, a recognizable logistic expression. The extinction probability of the process $\vec{N}$ is $\frac{\mu}{\lambda}$. For $\gamma > 0$ one has $u_1 < \frac{\mu}{\lambda}$, reflecting the fact that the tumor may be detected, or that it may issue a metastasis and then die out. See the anecdotes of Section 2.

To describe the combined distribution of the time τ of the first event and of the size of the primary at that time consider the mixte density-generating function

$$G_N(u, t) = \lim_{\epsilon \to 0} \frac{1}{\epsilon} E\, I(t \leq \tau < t+\epsilon)\, u^{N(t)}. \tag{4}$$

It is given by $\gamma u \frac{\partial}{\partial u} Q(u, t)$ and is equal to

$$G_N(u, t) = \gamma(u_2-u_1)^2 \frac{u \exp\{\beta t\}}{[(u_2-u)\exp\{\beta t\} + (u-u_1)]^2}. \tag{5}$$

From this one can obtain the generating function $\phi(u) = E\{u^{N(\tau)} | \tau < \infty\}$ of the size of tumor at time of first event given that such an event occurs.

It is

$$\phi(u) = \frac{(u_2-1)u}{u_2-u}, \tag{6}$$

a geometric distribution with expectation $1 + (u_2-1)^{-1}$ and variance $u_2(u_2-1)^{-2}$.

Now let us introduce a further assumption. (It is not quite right, but approximately correct.)

(A6). *The probability of discovery of the primary is not affected by the presence of metastases.*

Under this assumption, let $0 < v_1 < 1 < v_2$ be the roots of $\lambda v^2 - (\lambda+\mu+\gamma_2) v + \mu = 0$. Let

$$Q_2(v, t) = E\{v^{N(\tau+t)} \exp\{-\gamma_2 \int_\tau^{\tau+t} N(x)\, dx\} \mid \tau < \infty\}. \tag{7}$$

This is an expression similar to the $Q(u, t)$ used previously. The term $E\, v^{N(\tau+t)}$ can be interpreted as follows. It is the generating function of the primary size at time t after a first event, given that such an event occurred. The term $Q_2(1, t)$ represents the probability that, given an event occurred, the primary will be discovered at time t or more after the first event. Given the occurrence of a first event, the probability that it be the start of a metastasis is $\gamma_1(\gamma_1+\gamma_2)^{-1}$. Thus, letting T be the time elapsed between the start of a metastasis and the discovery of the primary, one has $Q_2(1, t) = P[T > t]$ conditionally on the fact that a first event occurred and that it was the start of a metastasis.

To simplify, let Ξ be the event that 1) a first event occurred, 2) it was the start of a metastasis, 3) the primary will eventually be discovered. Then, for the time T elapsed between the start of the metastasis and the discovery of the primary one has

$$F(t) = P[T \geq t \mid \Xi] = \frac{u_2 - v_1}{u_2(1-v_1)} [Q_2(1, t) - Q_2(1, \infty)] \tag{8}$$

Computation yields

$$F(t) = \frac{1 + A}{\exp\{\beta_2 t\} + A} \tag{9}$$

where

$$A = \frac{(u_2-v_2)}{(v_2-1)} \frac{(1-v_1)}{(u_2-v_1)} \tag{10}$$

and where $\beta_2 = \lambda(v_2-v_1) = [(\lambda-\mu)^2 + 2(\lambda+\mu)\gamma_2 + \gamma_2^2]^{1/2}$.

The size of the primary at discovery, given Ξ is given by the geometric distribution with generating function $(v_2-1)v(v_2-v)^{-1}$.

Now let us consider further what happens to the metastases. They grow as a birth and death process with coefficients λ_1 and μ_1. The equation $\lambda_1 w^2 - (\lambda_1+\mu_1)w + \mu_1 = 0$ has two roots $w_2 = 1$ and $w_1 = \frac{\mu_1}{\lambda_1}$. Let ξ be the time of discovery of the primary.

(A7). *Assume that the primary is removed at time ξ, so that it cannot issue metastases from ξ on. Count only those metastases issued from the primary, discounting the possibility that they may themselves metastasize.*

Then, the probability that no metastasis survived is

$$p = E \exp\{-\gamma_1(1-w_1) \int_0^\xi N(x) \, dx\}. \tag{11}$$

The surviving metastases have a Poisson distribution with an expectation $\gamma_1(1-w_1) \int_0^\xi N(x) \, dx$ given the process $\vec{N}$. From this one deduces that the number M of surviving metastases has a generating function

$$E z^M = \frac{\gamma_2}{\gamma_2 - \gamma_1(1-w_1)(z-1)} \tag{12}$$

and that

$$p = \frac{\gamma_2}{\gamma_2 + \gamma_1(1-w_1)} \tag{13}$$

The expected number of surviving metastases is $\frac{(1-w_1)\gamma_1}{\gamma_2}$.

We have assumed that the first metastasis issued grows according to a birth and death process with coefficients λ_1, μ_1. Let $\beta_3 = \lambda_1 - \mu_1$ and

$w_1 = \frac{\mu_1}{\lambda_1}$. For this first metastasis one can write an expression $E\, w^{M(t)} = Q_M(w, t)$ for the time t after the start of the metastasis. According to the same computation

$$Q_M(w, t) = w_1 + \frac{(1-w_1)(w-w_1)}{(1-w)\exp\{\beta_3 t\} + w - w_1}. \tag{14}$$

This may be rewritten in the form

$$Q_M(w, t) = \frac{(x-1)w_1}{x-w_1} + \frac{x(1-w_1)}{(x-w_1)} \frac{[(x-w_1)-(x-1)]w}{[(x-w_1)-(x-1)w]}, \tag{15}$$

exhibiting the geometric distribution with generating function $(1-y)(1-yw)^{-1}$ with $y = (x-1)(x-w_1)^{-1}$ and $x = \exp\{\beta_3 t\}$.

Now, conditionally on the event Ξ, the metastasis will have age T at time of discovery of the primary. Thus, conditionally on Ξ, the size $M = M(T)$ of that first metastasis has the generating function $E\, w^{M(T)} = E\, Q_M(w, T) = -\int Q_M(w, t)\, dF(t)$, where $F(t) = P(T > t)$ is given by the formula (9).

This formula is not easily calculable unless one assumes that $\beta_2 = \beta_3$. This assumption means that the net rate of growth of the metastasis is somewhat larger than that of the primary. That is not entirely an unreasonable assumption.

This leads to the following assertion.

Lemma 1. Assume that (A1) to (A6) hold and that $\beta_2 = \beta_3$. Then, conditionally on event Ξ, the size M of the first metastasis at discovery of the primary has a generating function

$$E\, w^M = \int_1^\infty \frac{(x-1)w_1}{(x-w_1)} \frac{(1+A)}{(x+A)^2}\, dx$$

$$+ \int_1^\infty \frac{x(1-w_1)}{(x-w_1)} \frac{(1-w_1)w}{[(x-w_1)-(x-1)w]} \frac{1+A^-}{(x+A)^2}\, dx, \tag{16}$$

where $A = (u_2 - v_2)(v_2 - 1)^{-1}(1 - v_1)(u_2 - v_1)^{-1}$.

These integrals could be evaluated. We shall not do so, but note only that the geometric distribution involved under the integral sign is one with generating function $(1-y)w(1-yw)^{-1}$ where the variable $y = (x-1)(x-w_1)^{-1}$ has a density

$$f(y) = \frac{1-D}{(1-Dy)^2} \tag{17}$$

for $0 < y < 1$ and for $D = \dfrac{A+w_1}{A+1}$.

One could obtain further expressions. A particular one refers to variables analogous to those discussed in [2], but referring only to the time elapsed between discovery of the primary and discovery of the *first born* metastasis.

Here it is probably not too unrealistic to assume that during the time between the start of the metastasis and the discovery of the primary, nobody will look for the metastasis and it will not be discovered. (This is not quite true; see anecdotes in Section 2.)

One could also assume that the discovery process is similar to that of the primary so that if the size of the metastasis is $M(t)$ at t the probability of discovery in $(t, t+h]$ is $\gamma_3 M(t) h + o(h)$.

Condition on Ξ. Let r_1 and r_2 be the roots of $\lambda_1 r^2 - [\lambda_1+\mu_1+\gamma_3]r + \mu_1 = 0$, with $r_1 < r_2$. Let S be the time elapsed between the discovery of the primary and the discovery of the first born metastasis. Then, assuming as above that $\beta_2 = \beta_3$ and letting $\beta_4 = \lambda_1(r_2-r_1)$ one can compute that

$$P(S>s) = w_1 + (1-w_1)\frac{H}{H-A}\{1 + \frac{1+A}{H-A}\log(\frac{1+A}{1+H})\} \tag{18}$$

where

$$H = \frac{r_1-w_1}{1-r_1} + \frac{(1-w_1)(r_2-r_1)}{(1-r_1)(r_2-1)}\frac{1}{\exp\{\beta_4 s\}-1}. \tag{19}$$

We shall not use this formula, for two reasons. One is that it refers only to the time S of observation of the first metastasis and is therefore not quite comparable to the times used in [2]. This is not too serious, however, since most of the cases discussed in [2] had only one metastasis. The second reason is more serious. After discovery of the primary, the patient is subjected to a type of screening entirely different from the casual inspection accorded by doctors to presumably healthy individuals. One could compensate for some of that by taking γ_3 much larger than γ_2. However, that would not do. Typically, the patient will be given a thorough check at the time of discovery of the primary. Thereafter he will have periodic check ups, once a month for perhaps a year or half a year. Then the check ups will be less frequent, occurring perhaps every three months for a couple of years. Then they will be even less frequent, tapering out to less than the often recommended annual check up after five or six years.

The distribution of the time of discovery of the metastasis may be grossly influenced by the observation process, at least for slow growing metastases. Thus, it seems too perilous to take a chance on studies of variables such as S unless the observations are part of a highly controlled experiment.

4. The Heterogeneity of Patients

In Section 2 we have recalled certain studies on doubling times of tumors. The observed doubling times do indeed vary considerably. To apply the formulas of Section 3 to a group of patients it seems imperative to take such differences into account. This could be done, for instance, by assuming that the coefficients $\lambda-\mu$ and $\lambda_1-\mu_1$ of Section 3 vary according to a certain lognormal distribution. A different type of assumption would be that each patient proceeds according to his own time, related to calendar in an increasing manner, but otherwise fairly arbitrary.

Now note that several of the expressions given in Section 3 are actually independent of the time scale used. By this we mean the following.

Suppose that the "time" t involved in the assumptions (A1) to (A7) is not calendar time but that t is an increasing function $t = h(t_c)$ of the true calendar time t_c.

Let h be such that $h(t') = 0$ for some t' and such that $\lim h(t_c) = \infty$ as $t_c \to \infty$. Then, formulas (6), (10), (12), (13), (15), (16) and (17) remain entirely valid. Therefore, these formulas remain applicable to a group of patients as long as the roots u_i and v_i and the ratios $\frac{\gamma_1}{\gamma_2}$ remain constant from patient to patient. The time scale h can vary arbitrarily from patient to patient. In particular the "doubling times" can have any distribution they please. The roots u_i depend only on the ratio $\frac{\mu}{\lambda}$ and on the ratio $\frac{(\gamma_1+\gamma_2)}{\lambda}$. Similarly the v_i are functions of $\frac{\mu}{\lambda}$ and $\frac{\gamma_2}{\lambda}$. The term w_1 is of course just $\frac{\mu_1}{\lambda_1}$. Lemma 1 does involve the assumption $\beta_2 = \beta_3$, that is $(\lambda_1-\mu_1)^2 = (\lambda-\mu)^2 + 2(\lambda+\mu)\gamma_2 + \gamma_2^2$.

We shall argue that the system is not compatible with experience even if that supplementary assumption is not closely satisfied.

Of course, one can readily expect that a ratio such as $\frac{\mu}{\lambda}$, which represents the percentage of cell loss in the tumor, will vary from tumor to tumor. Some of the calculations given below would still be valid if $\frac{\lambda}{\mu}$ varies moderately. They would force $\frac{\mu_1}{\lambda_1}$ in an unacceptable range. The ratio $\frac{\mu}{\lambda}$ has been studied experimentally through experiments involving labeled thymidine incorporation. An estimate, for sarcomas, is $\frac{\mu}{\lambda} = .40$. (See [8], Table 6.2.)

The situation for the ratio $\frac{\gamma_1}{\gamma_2}$ is more touchy. The term γ_1 refers to an instantaneous probability of release of a metastatic cell, while γ_2 refers to probability of discovery of the primary. This means that perhaps $\frac{\gamma_1}{\gamma_2}$ varies in fairly wide range. However, we shall argue below assuming that all these ratios are kept constant and try to guess at possible numerical values for them.

One first observation is that, even if a person is under a fairly good medical scrutiny, a tumor is rarely observable until it reaches a size equivalent to about 10^9 cells. The expected size at discovery being $(v_2-1)^{-1}$, this means that the order of magnitude of v_2-1 is

$$v_2 - 1 \sim 10^{-9} \tag{20}$$

Taking $\lambda = 1$ for simplicity, we can write

$$v_2 = \frac{1+\mu+\gamma_2}{2} + \tfrac{1}{2}[(1-\mu)^2 + 2\gamma_2(1+\mu) + \gamma_2^2]^{1/2}. \tag{21}$$

Thus, in such a framework γ_2 will be very small and a Taylor expansion gives the approximation

$$v_2 - 1 \sim \gamma_2 \, [\tfrac{1}{2} + \frac{1+\mu}{1-\mu}]. \tag{22}$$

This would go for any form of solid tumor. To proceed further, we shall refer to osteosarcoma and take certain numbers which seem to be fairly consistent with many observations.

One of the numbers is the percentage of patients who have already detectable metastatic disease at the time of discovery of the primary. This is a number q with value of the order of .14 (one out of seven or more). Assuming that Lemma 1 holds and that discoverable size is n, this means that $P[M \geqslant n]$ in Lemma 1 must be sizable, say about .10.

Now in Lemma 1, one has

$$P[M \geqslant n] = (1-w_1) \int_0^1 \left(\frac{x-1}{x-w_1}\right) y^n f(y) \, dy \tag{23}$$

with $f(y) = (1-D)(1-Dy)^{-2}$. Thus

$$P(M \geqslant n) \leqslant \frac{1-w_1}{1-D} \frac{1}{n+1} + \frac{1}{n(n+1)} \tag{24}$$

Now $(1-D) = (1-w_1)(A+1)^{-1}$. Thus for a detectable size n we get

$$P(M \geqslant n) = \frac{1}{n+1}\left[A+1+\frac{1}{n}\right]. \tag{25}$$

One concludes that, for a frequency q of presence of detectable metastases at time of discovery of the primary, one should have $(A+1) \geqslant qn$.

This argument relies on the validity of Lemma 1, and hence on the equality $\beta_2 = \beta_3$ which gives the particular density f used here. However, similar inequalities could be derived for a variety of other densities f.

Two other observable quantities are 1) the proportion p of patients who never develop metastases and 2) the total number of metastases ever found. The value of p is of the general order of .20 or perhaps even a little higher. Thus equation (13) suggests the approximate equality $\gamma_2 \sim (.20)[\gamma_2 + \gamma_1(1-w_1)]$ or equivalently

$$\frac{\gamma_1(1-w_1)}{\gamma_2} \sim 4. \tag{26}$$

If the (.20) is not deemed accurate one could use $\gamma_1(1-w_1)\gamma_2^{-1} = (1-p)p^{-1}$. It will be seen below that the fact that both p and q are nonnegligible is enough to create some trouble. Now, let us pass to the evaluation of the coefficient A. According to formula (10) one has $A = (u_2-v_2)(v_2-1)^{-1}(1-v_1)(u_2-v_1)^{-1} \leqslant (u_2-v_2)(v_2-1)^{-1}$. Using formula (25) with $q \sim .1$ and $n \sim 10^9$ one sees that A should be of the general order of magnitude 10^8 or at least 10^7 if detection can be carried out for 10^8 cells. Since (v_2-1) is of the order 10^{-9}, this would imply $u_2 - v_2 \geqslant 10^{-1}$ or, in the extreme case, $u_2 - v_2 \geqslant 10^{-2}$. For values in that range Taylor's formula (22) is still approximately valid, leading to the approximate equality $\frac{(u_2-v_2)}{v_2-1} \sim \frac{\gamma_1}{\gamma_2}$. Thus we are led to the conclusion that A and therefore $\frac{\gamma_1}{\gamma_2}$ must be about 10^8 or 10^7 but that $\frac{\gamma_1(1-w_1)}{\gamma_2}$ must be about 4. In other words $(1-w_1)$ should be about $4 \cdot 10^{-8}$ or at best $4 \cdot 10^{-7}$.

Since $(1-w_1) = \dfrac{(\lambda_1 - \mu_1)}{\lambda_1}$ is the excess of birth over death probabilities in the metastasis, a value $(1-w_1) = 4\ 10^{-7}$ or even 10^{-6} is not reasonable. We have mentioned above that for sarcomas $1-w_1$ is about .6. For certain carcinomas it may be about $4\ 10^{-2}$, but the value obtained here is off by a factor of 10^5 or 10^4. This argument does not take into account the fact that there may be several metastases. However it would take an unreasonably large number of them to make it totally invalid.

We have used the probability p of not developing any metastases, according to formula (13), Section 3. One could also use the total expected number m of metastases (arising from the primary). According to formula (12), m is also $\dfrac{\gamma_1(1-w_1)}{\gamma_2}$. A value of $m = 4$ is not unreasonable.

Another view of the matter can be obtained by looking at the distribution F of equation 9. If the probability p of remaining metastasis free is of the order of .20, this equation implies that the time elapsed between the first metastatic event and the discovery of the primary, is of the order of 2 or 3 doubling times for the primary. Thus, unless the metastases grow extremely fast compared to the primary, they will not be detectable at the time the primary is discovered.

If any such argument is at all valid one may ask what is wrong with the assumptions of the model. It does rely on the "primarily exponential" growth of the tumors. It also relies on the assumption that probability of discovery of a tumor and probability of release of a metastasis are both proportional to the tumor size. Some authors prefer to use a probability of metastatic events proportional to the 2/3 power of the tumor volume. This would imply that metastatic events occur comparatively earlier than they do in the present model and might lead to different answers. Unfortunately the mathematical derivations become rather complex. There is not much evidence for the proportionality-to-2/3-power idea. It comes from the misconception that a tumor is like a ball having contact with the rest of the body only through its surface. The tumor area depends strongly on its shape which may be far from spherical. It may be entirely in contact with the rest of the body through ordinary capillaries and tumor "sinusoids". It may invade local veins.

We have already observed that variation of our coefficient $\frac{\gamma_1}{\gamma_2}$ from patient to patient is a definite possibility.

As an extreme case one may suppose that not all tumors shed metastasis producing cells, either because they do not shed, or because the immune system prevents the survival of cells once shed. This may explain away part of the difficulties. However some remain.

Let us forget about the assumption that metastases are born according to the process described by Assumption (A4) and consider instead an arbitrary random time τ defined by the past of the process $N(t)$ up to $t = \tau$. Interpret this time as the time of birth of a metastasis.

Let T be the time elapsed between the birth of the metastasis and the discovery of the primary, conditionally upon this discovery.

One can write, conditionally on knowledge of the process N up to τ,

$$P[T \geq t] = \frac{[G(t)]^{N(\tau)} - v_1^{N(\tau)}}{1 - v_1^{N(\tau)}} \tag{27}$$

with

$$G(t) = v_1 + \frac{(v_2 - v_1)(1 - v_1)}{(v_2 - 1)\exp\{\beta_2 t\} + (1 - v_1)} \tag{28}$$

From this one can find the median and other quantiles of T and ascertain the probable size of the metastasis at discovery of the primary. It turns out that if β_2 and β_3 are about equal, in order to have a sizable chance of seeing a metastasis at discovery of the primary one would have to start it when $N(\tau)$ is rather small, of the order of a few hundreds. This can be seen easily without much computation in another way. (It is a deterministic way, but a solidly established birth and death process is almost deterministic.)

The assumption that the primary is detected at a size about 10^9 means that it has lived through 30 doubling times. The assumption that a metastasis is detected at about $(1.3)\,10^8$ means that it went through 27 of its doubling times. If one claims that the doubling time of the primary is 1.35 times that of the metastasis (a purely gratuitous assumption), this means that the metastasis was born when the primary had gone through 10 doubling times and had a size about 10^3.

Thus, unless i) some tumors do not shed metastases and others do and ii) the metastases grow much more rapidly than the primary, the metastasis must be born when the primary was very young.

This conclusion goes in the same directions as the findings of (2). However, in the present case one cannot possibly conceive of "new primaries" since osteoid (bone matrix) producing cells in the lung cannot originate there.

There are various other possibilities. One is that the metastases are born from clumps of cells detached from the primary. There is some evidence that such clumps have a better chance of adhering to a capillary wall and of starting a growing birth and death process. However, i) tumor cells do not adhere well to each other, and ii) the size of the clumps must be fairly small. The evidence for the second assertion is meager, but there is some. Screening of blood samples after surgery yields mostly single circulating cancer cells. Also the metastases occur mostly in the capillary beds of the outer portion of the lungs. So the clumps must be small enough to get there. However if the cells are shed in clumps of about 10^3 cells (approximately 10^{-1} mm diameter), metastases would be detectable at diagnosis of the primary if they are born when the size of the primary was around 10^5 (if $\beta_2 = \beta_3$) or perhaps up to 10^8 (if $\beta_3 = 1.35\,\beta_2$). The trouble with such an explanation is that clumps of size 10^3 are about 10^2 times too big to fit in the accepted descriptions of the cell shedding process. However, it may be a possibility. See [3].

There is also the possibility that the cells are dislodged into the blood stream as a result of trauma or other events in a manner essentially independent of the size of the primary.

Finally, even though there is insufficient available data on this aspect of the situation, one may conjecture that the cells are released by a process entirely different from that covered by assumption (A4). In (A4) cells are released singly at random times. For patients with multiple pulmonary metastases, the sizes are often comparable, leading to the suspicion that they may be of similar age. In other cases, there may be several of one size, say 10^9, and many of a much smaller size, say 10^8. thus one might conceive of the possibility that cells are released in groups (but not adherent to each other) at the occurrence of trauma or other events. In the early stages of osteosarcoma the young patients are ordinarily very active. The possibility, although very conjectural, seems to deserve further study.

Another possibility is that the growth of the primary is not all representable by a birth and death process. It may be very irregular. As mentioned linear birth and death processes look almost like deterministic exponential growth when established. There have been claims that many tumors grow according to the so-called cube-root growth pattern (see [8]). This means that the diameter of the tumor increases linearly in time. One may be able to achieve patterns of this general type by introducing non-linear effects in the birth and death processes.

5. References

1) R. Bartoszyński, B. W. Brown, C. M. McBride and J. R. Thompson, "Some nonparametric techniques for estimating the intensity function of a cancer related nonstationary Poisson process". To appear *Ann. Statist.*

2) R. Bartoszyński, B. W. Brown, J. R. Thompson, "Metastatic and Systemic factors in Neoplastic progression". Preprint, March 1981. Chapter in this volume.

3) Isaiah J. Fidler, Douglas M. Gersten and Ian R. Hart, "The biology of cancer invasion and metastasis" *Advances in Cancer Research. Vol. 28* pp. 149-250. (1978).

4) W. L. Joseph, D. L. Morton, P. C. Atkins, "Prognostic significance of tumor doubling time in evaluating operability in pulmonary metastatic disease". *The Journal of Thoracic and Cardiovascular Surgery, Vol. 61 #1*, Jan. 1971, pp. 23-32.

5) A. W. Pearlman, "Breast Cancer Influence of growth in prognosis and treatment evaluation". *Cancer, Vol. 38*, pp. 1826-1833 (1976).

6) P. S. Puri, "A class of stochastic models of response after infection in the absence of defense mechanism". *Proc. Fifth Berkeley Symposium on Math. Stat. and Proba. Vol IV*, pp. 511-535. Univ. of Calif. Press, Berkeley, 1967.

7) J. S. Spratt, T. L. Spratt, "Rate of growth of pulmonary metastases and host survival". *Ann. Surgery, Vol. 159*, #2, pp. 161-171 (1964).

8) G. G. Steel, *Growth Kinetics of Tumor*, Clarendon Press, Oxford 351 pp. (1977).

6. Discussion by R. Bartoszyński, B. W. Brown and J. R. Thompson

We thank Professor LeCam for his elegant argument and provocative comments although we are (not surprisingly) not in total agreement with all of the later.

LeCam argues that an exponentially growing tumor system in which the probability of detection of the tumor and the probability of issuing a metastasis is proportional to tumor size is incompatible with some simple observable facts. Due to the exponential process, the time window for detection is narrow. In particular, about 0.87 of all tumors should be detected within about three doubling times of the tumor. The assumption about metastasis implies that about the same proportion of all metastases should be emitted in the same time period. It takes metastases a long time to grow to detectable size. (For illustration, one might consider tumor doubling time of about two months and time to detection of five years.) If a sizable proportion of patients present with detectable metastasis, the tumor must be very prone to metastasis so that even small tumors have a very high probability of metastasizing. But this would mean that almost all patients would sooner or later have metastases discovered which is contrary to actual experience.

This is a good argument. After much data analysis, we concluded that an exponentially growing tumor system in which the probability of detection of the tumor and the probability of issuing a metastasis is proportional to tumor size is incompatible with fairly complex clinical data.

After arriving at a similar conclusion for differing reasons, we differ from Professor LeCam on the next step. He conjectures "wild heterogeneity" and decides that modeling must be abandoned. This seems an extreme reaction. Our approach was to modify the model. We added a "systemic" factor to the metastatic process. (Incidentally, the interpretation of this factor as "spontaneous new primaries" is LeCam's. We were purposely careful not to speculate on the nature of this process.) This factor increased the heterogeneity of the time of first metastasis. With this factor included we obtained what we consider an acceptable fit to at least one set of clinical data.

The methods used in the modeling accounted for the proportion who did not develop metastases during the observation process. However we do not use the proportion who present with metastasis. The primary reason for this is that we are interested in using the model to examine many sets of data available to us at M. D. Anderson. This institution is a referral center only, consequently, the mixture of patients which is seen depends not only on the natural history of the disease but on the decision of primary care physicians as to who warrants referral. Consequently, there is probably a substantial bias in stage at presentation (as compared to global experience). However, one might assume that metastases which have had four or more years to grow would be detectable at the time of treatment of the primary. Noting that our estimated median time to detection of the primary is five years, we look at Table 1 and estimate that perhaps 3.5 percent of patients should have detectable metastases at diagnosis. From report 4 of End Results in Cancer, we find that 4 percent of the 25698 diagnoses of breast cancer examined from 1955 to 1964 were metastatic at presentation.

Professor LeCam concludes: "Thus it seems too perilous to take a chance on studies of variables such as S (metastasis observation time) unless the observations are part of a highly controlled experiment." The heterogeneities inevitable in clinical data sets are always a problem. But if we disdain to use such data in favor of in vitro or anecdotal experience, we will be rather like the little boy who insisted on searching for his dime under the bright street light rather than in the dark alley where he lost it. Only by speculative clinical data based modeling can we bring on line the potentially useful data streams which can lead to a greater understanding of the whys and wherefores of cancer. Almost all data is collected in the first place in the light of an explicit or implicit model. If our work in metastatic modeling achieves nothing else, it will have brought into the consciousness of a number of clinicians the fact that a good record of metastasis times might be a reasonable thing to keep.

7. Reply by Lucien Le Cam

My distinguished colleagues have raised several points which would need lengthy elaboration. I shall only respond to one.

It should be clear from their comments and from my paper that I have trouble understanding what they mean by a "systemic effect", distinct from the metastatic process but leading to neoplastic growth. I was peripherally involved in a study which showed, among other things, that the ultrastructure of normal cells near a tumor, but not touching it, is somewhat intermediate between "normal" and "cancerous". There are publications to this effect in the biological literature. However the evidence is far from conclusive. Tumors of epithelial nature have been known to "recruit" fibroblasts "touching" them, but that is a different story.

The fact that my colleagues obtained a decent fit by adding a systemic component to the metastatic one does not mean that they have thereby obtained a correct explanation, or the only possible one. To obtain a check one should first eliminate from the data those tumors that are demonstrably metastases.

Pathologists can determine if a liver or bone tumor arose from a mammary adenocarcinoma. In the case of osteosarcoma mentioned in my paper, this is quite simple. It would be very unusual for a pulmonary cell to decide to produce osteoid. Assuming that after all demonstrably metastatic events have been removed there would remain unexplained neoplasms, further studies would be needed.

In this author's opinion fitting distributions of occurrence is unlikely to produce a clear cut answer since the distributions are affected by very many factors on which our information is poor.

However, and contrary to what my colleagues imply, I do agree with them that one should continue to study the matter, mathematically and otherwise.

Optimal Multiple Decision Problems: Some Principles and Procedures Applicable in Cancer Drug Screening

Robert Bohrer

University of Illinois at Urbana

ABSTRACT

This paper exemplifies how both the user of statistics and the statistician must care in deciding, together, the goals of their statistical analyses. Examples are cited wherein similar goals lead to very different optimal solutions, wherein different goals lead to similar optimal solutions, and where the natural optimality criterion leads to unnatural multiple decision rules. The principles and procedures discussed, which are applicable quite generally, are viewed from the applied problem of drug screening.

1. Why Optimal Rules?

One might ask why much effort should be devoted to finding best statistical procedures, especially in cases where common sense or other guides might supply seemingly reasonable procedures. There are several answers to this question.

First, to seek a best procedure requires the statistician and the researcher for whom he works to define carefully their idea of what they mean by a good procedure. Second, and closely related, is the fact (see, e.g., Sections 2 and 3) that two closely related criteria of goodness can lead to very different statistical procedures having very different statistical

---

This research was funded by the National Science Foundation Grant MCS-79-02581.

properties.

Also, common sense rules can, in some cases, behave very badly. See, for example, [12], [15], and [5].

Moreover, even a good, common sense procedure can sometimes be beaten by an order of magnitude. Suppose, for example, that the life, X, of an experimental animal is at least T (an unknown parameter) and, thereafter, is an exponential random variable, having probability density function $f(x) = \exp(T-x)$ if $x > T$ (and $f(x) = 0$ otherwise). On the basis of n random samples of such lifetimes, the "natural" estimator for expected life is the sample average, which is unbiased with variance $1/n$. On the other hand, if one seeks minimum variance unbiased estimators, it can be shown that a better and, in fact, best estimator is $Y + (1 - 1/n)$, where Y is the smallest of the observed lifetimes; the variance of this alternative unbiased estimator is $\frac{1}{n^2}$, an order of magnitude better than the sample average.

2. Which-sided tests?

Wherein closely related criteria give very different procedures. Suppose we want the most powerful test possible for testing how a drug treatment compares with no treatment in increase (or decrease) of expected life, $E(X)$. On the basis of n observed life extensions, assumed, for simplicity, to be normal with known variance, two most powerful tests of significance level .05 for the null hypothesis of no effect are to reject if the sample average is too small or, alternatively, to reject if it is too large. The first test protects against too-quick adoption of the drug, while the second protects against discarding a drug too readily. For example, if the drug is exactly as good as nothing, then the first test would decide it is effective only 5% of the time, while the second would accept its effectiveness 95% of the time. In such a case, where the consequences of the decision are so different, it is critical for the drug screener and statistician to decide clearly which protection is to be guaranteed by their optimality criterion.

3. The case of the missing labels:

Wherein, again, two very similar criteria lead to two very different procedures. Here is a hypothetical example in which a physician has supplies of two drugs, one of which is effective with probability .50365 and the other with probability .1864. Unfortunately, the labels distinguishing the two drugs have been lost, and the physician must determine, as well as possible, which drug is the more effective. If "as well as possible" means by observing the drug effects on as few patients as possible, then [2] shows that sampling should be done with the drug which, at any point in time, is maximum likelihood estimator for the worse drug. On the other hand, if it means maximizing the number of patients in the screen who receive the more effective drug, then Feldman [9] shows that exactly the other drug should be given. Here, again, the applicator must decide which of the two optimality criteria is preferable, or even usable, in the problem at hand.

4. Multiple decision rules.

The author's attention for the past few years has been directed to problems wherein one needs to decide which of several parameters, e.g., drugs, are positive and which are negative. The problem of multiple comparisons is that, if the decision about each parameter has chance $1 - \alpha$ of being correct, then the expected number of incorrect decisions about the n parameters is αn. For example, one expects one out of twenty 95% confidence intervals not to cover. One must determine the price to be paid in order to be as confident as required about all one's inferences simultaneously. And, on the other side of this coin, one might be able to use possible dependencies among the inferences to good advantage.

The multiple decision problem considered here is to maximize (in some sense) the expected number of correct decisions made, subject to

$$P(no\ misclassifications) \geqslant 1 - \alpha \qquad (1)$$

or a corresponding bound on the (closely related) expected number of errors made. Almost all of the salient ideas are captured in the case of classifying just two parameters, to which most subsequent attention is devoted.

5. Testing for better or no-better:

Wherein the optimal rule incriminates the optimality criterion. One approach to the problem of real interest, i. e., that of section 6, is less unwieldy when reduced as follows. It illustrates a useful technique while, in this case, the details do not obscure the idea of what goes wrong, as much as in the corresponding case of Section 6. Suppose that improvements of two drugs over a control are independent random variables, X_i ($i = 1, 2$) having the normal $N(M_i, 1)$ distribution. Consider decision rules of the form $D_i(X_1, X_2) = 0$ or 1 according as we decide that drug i is no-better or better than the control on observing (X_1, X_2). As our optimality criterion, we seek to maximize, over all $M_i > d$, the minimum expected number of correct decisions, subject to $P_0[\text{no incorrect decisions}] = 1 - \alpha$. Denoting the $N(0, 1)$ density by g and the $N(d, 1)$ density by g^*, one might proceed by considering the worst better case, $M_i = d$ for $i = 1, 2$, and to maximize the risk, i.e., the integral of

$$[D_1 + D_2] g^* - k (1-D_1)(1-D_2) g, \tag{2}$$

where k is chosen to satisfy (1).

Inspection of (2) shows that whenever either drug is judged better than the control, the k-term is 0, so that the other drug can be judged positive also "at no extra cost". One thus judges either both drugs as equal to or both as better than the control, the latter being the decision if $X_1 + X_2 > k^*$, where k^* is chosen to satisfy (1).

However, this is a silly rule, since it does not allow the decision that one drug is better and the other is no better. When this is, in fact, the true state of nature, with the good drug being extremely good, then one will decide nearly all the time that the worthless drug is good, even if its X_i value is negative. The "optimal" decision rule incriminates itself by this review of its potential bad performance. The problem is that what we thought was what we meant by optimal was wrong, since it did not have a risk contribution from cases where one drug is better and the other no better than the control. With a more realistic risk function, this approach would be potentially useful, both here and in the problem of Section 6, although the author has tried it at considerable length with little reward.

6. Testing for better or for worse: several maximum rules

In this case, one is required to decide, subject to (1), which of several parameters (drugs) are better and which are worse than a control. This sounds very much like the problem of the previous section. However, it differs in requiring the detection of substandard parameters. In practice, for example, the analogue to Dunnett's [8] rule for use in Section 5 is shown to be too liberal by Appendix A2 in [4].

For (at least) definiteness and for application of he tables below, the "usual" assumptions are made. Namely, estimators, $\hat{\theta}_i$, for the two parameters θ_i (i = 1, 2) are available. These are normally distributed with mean θ_i, variance V, and correlation ρ. Independent of the $\hat{\theta}_i$ is the variance estimator $\hat{V}$, such that $n\hat{V}/V$ is a chi-square random variable with n degrees of freedom. For example, this is the case in usual analysis of variance situations, viz., when equal numbers of observations are taken on each of two drugs under study and where a (possibly different) number are taken with the control. If the control performance is known, then no observations on it are needed, and $\rho = 0$, whereas, if equal numbers are taken on the two drugs and control and if $\hat{\theta}_i$ is the difference in sample means of drug i and the control, then $\rho = .5$. If more observations are taken on the control, so that, for the fixed total sample size, $var(\hat{\theta}_i)$ is minimized, then $\rho = \sqrt{2} - 1 = .414$.

Consider first the problem of classifying only the one parameter, θ_1. The fundamental lemma of Neyman and Pearson shows that the best two-decision (+ or −) rule decides that θ_1 is positive only in case $\hat{\theta}_1 > 0$ and negative if $\hat{\theta}_i < 0$. However, this rule misclassifies parameter values near 0 with probability .5. If α, in (1) is, as usual, less than .5, no such two-decision rules suffices. For two or more parameters, the situation is even worse.

The way to achieve (1) is to permit, in addition to + and -, the decision "0", meaning that the the data are inconclusive about the parameter in question. In fact, Bahadur [1] shows how a t-statistic can be used to make optimal decisions about a single parameter in this case, avoiding the troubles cited in [12], [15], and [5].

6.1. The Spjøtvoll (Sp) Cross, [6].

What can be done for the case of deciding the signs of two or more parameters? In [3] and [4], multiple t-statistics are employed to decide about the parameters. In the case of two parameters, such a rule subdivides the $(\hat{\theta}_1, \hat{\theta}_2)$-plane into the nine regions shown in Figure 1A, where, for example, if the estimator-pair falls into the square containing the origin, then one decides that the data are inconclusive about both parameters, while if it falls in the upper, right-hand corner, then both parameters are decided to be positive.

The probability of correct classification for this rule is seen in [3] to be a non-central t probability which increases to unity as the magnitude of the true parameter-value increases. In fact, in [3], the work of Spjotvoll is used to prove this multiple t-statistic, "Spjøtvoll Cross" to be optimal in the following sense. Among rules which have the same or smaller expected number of incorrect decisions, the Spjøtvoll cross maximizes the minimum expected number of correct classifications. This minimum is achieved in the limit as all parameter values approach 0. In the case of two parameters, the region on which no misclassifications are made if both $\hat{\theta}_i$ are positive is shown in Figure 1B, while the region of estimators for which a correct decision is made about $\hat{\theta}_1$ is shown in Figure 1C. The second column of Table 1 gives the expected numbers of correct classifications for this Sp cross, achieving (1) with $\alpha = .05$ and variance known.

Of course, to implement this rule in practice, the width of the "arms" of the Sp cross must be determined. This is the problem to which most of the fun of [3] and [4] is devoted.

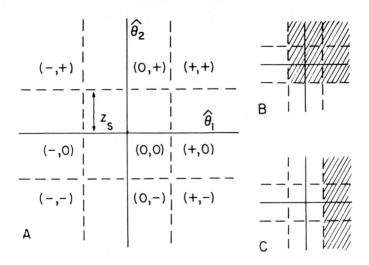

Fig. 1. The Sp cross. (A) The nine decision regions. (B) The region where no incorrect decisions are made if $\theta_1, \theta_2 > 0$. (C) The region where correct decision is made about θ_1 if $\theta_1 > 0$.

6.2. The Celtic Cross, [6].

Can one improve on the Sp cross if the error criterion is (1), rather than bounding the expected number of errors? The two error measures are bound, by the likes of the Bonferroni inequality, to be close together. On the other hand, one might suspect that in cases where one parameter, and its estimator, are extremely large, the one-decision arms of the cross might not need to be wider than the α-point of the $\hat{\theta}_i$ distribution. In fact, an argument of epsilons and deltas shows that if the one-decision arms are decreased by ϵ and the no-decision region increased by the δ necessary to maintain (1), then the minimum number of correct decisions is increased. This process can be carried to the extreme mentioned above, with the resulting region in the shape of a Celtic cross, pictured in Figure 2, and expected numbers of correct decisions given in Table 1. Subject to the convexity property of Section 6.3, the Celtic cross gives minimax correct classifications among rules satisfying (1) with rectangular no-decision regions.

Table 1. Expected Number of Correct Classifications
For Four Rules at Different Parameter Pairs, (θ_1, θ_2)
(Data for the SP, Celtic, and DC Crosses are Reproduced from [6].)

A) $\rho = .5$

(θ_1, θ_2)	D.C.	SP.	Celtic	A.C.
(-4,0)	1.0255	1.0043	1.0258	.99040
(-3,0)	.8714	.8759	.8797	.8960
(-2,0)	.5044	.5410	.5251	.5788
(-1,0)	.1708	.1936	.1826	.2020
(0,0)	.0500	.0500	.0500	.0500
(1,0)	.1831	.1936	.1945	.2256
(2,0)	.5254	.5410	.5446	.6212
(3,0)	.8809	.8759	.8921	.9443
(4,0)	1.0270	1.0043	1.0287	1.0393

B) $\rho = .4$

(θ_1, θ_2)	D.C.	SP.	Celtic	A.C.
(-4,0)	1.0265	1.0043	1.0265	1.0378
(-3,0)	.8807	.8759	.8847	.9350
(-2,0)	.5224	.5410	.5331	.6073
(-1,0)	.1802	.1936	.1866	.2215
(0,0)	.0502	.0500	.0500	.0502
(1,0)	.1936	.1936	.1960	.1984
(2,0)	.5385	.5410	.5485	.5675
(3,0)	.8878	.8759	.8943	.8892
(4,0)	1.0276	1.0043	1.0287	.9915
(-4,4)	1.9814	1.9586	1.9814	1.9815
(-3,3)	1.8206	1.7018	1.8168	1.8246
(-2,2)	1.1744	1.0322	1.1476	1.2734
(-1,1)	.3276	.3372	.3330	.4649
(0,0)	.0502	.0500	.0500	.0502
(1,1)	.3768	.3372	.3642	.2679
(2,2)	1.1590	1.0322	1.1306	.7702
(3,3)	1.7974	1.7018	1.7850	1.3866
(4,4)	1.9798	1.9586	1.9786	1.8312

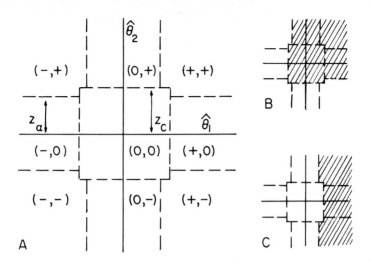

Fig. 2. The Celtic cross. (A) The nine decision regions. (B) The region where no incorrect decisions are made if $\theta_1, \theta_2 > 0$. (C) The region where correct decision is made about θ_1 if $\theta_1 > 0$.

6.3. The Double Cross (DC): an Optimal Solution from Linear Programming, [6].

Considering the requirements of a maximin solution subject to (1), one wants to maximize the probability, in the limit as the parameters approach 0, of the two adjacent two-decision regions plus the one-decision region, subject to the sum of probabilities of the no-decision region plus two one-decision regions plus the proper two-decision being at least $1 - \alpha$. These conditions define a linear programming problem from which to solve for the chances of the nine regions of the $(\hat{\theta}_1, \hat{\theta}_2)$-plane. There are, in fact, two solutions, when the rules are required to have the following natural convexity property:

> If an estimator-pair is in a two decision region and if either estimator is increased in magnitude, then the resulting estimator-pair is in the same two-decision region.

The Double Cross, pictured in Figure 3 and evaluated in Table 1, is investigated in [6]. The DC is seen to be marginally better in expected correct classifications in the limit at $(0, 0)$, as its optimality assures, and to

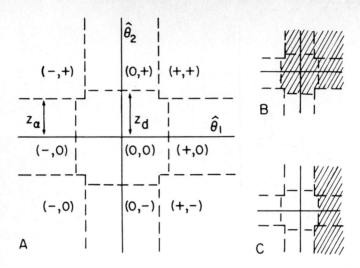

Fig. 3. The D. C. (A) The nine decision regions. (B) The region where no incorrect decisions are made if $\theta_1, \theta_2 > 0$. (C) The region where correct decision is made about θ_1 if $\theta_1 > 0$.

be competitive with, if not better than, the Sp and Celtic crosses at other $(\hat{\theta}_1, \hat{\theta}_2)$ values. Unfortunately, the DC is shown to violate (1) for parameters $(0-, \theta_2)$ as θ_2 approaches infinity. However, computations indicate that no violation of occurs for θ_2 less than 4 standard deviations away from 0 (in the known variance case); thus, for all practical, if not theoretical, purposes, the DC satisfies (1).

6.4. The Arrow Cross (AC): a Truly Optimal Rule?

As noted, but not investigated, in [6] and above, there is a second solution to the linear programming problem of finding a maximin solution. For this solution, both two-decision regions have the same probability, β (say), which is the smaller $P(\hat{\theta}_i > z_\alpha, i=1, 2)$ and $P(\hat{\theta}_1 > z_\alpha, \hat{\theta}_2 < -z_\alpha)$, where z_α is the upper α point of the $\hat{\theta}_i$ distribution. One way to achieve this is (for $\rho > 0$) by taking the $(+,+)$ region to be $[\hat{\theta}_i > z_B, i = 1, 2]$, where z_B is as large as this requires. To guarantee (1), the no-decision region is, as pictured in Figure 4, the union of four squares. The squares in quadrants 2 and 4 have side z_α, while the side, z_c, in quadrants 1 and 3

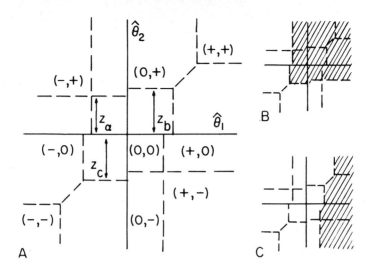

Fig. 4. The A. C. (A)(B)(C) as in Fig's. 1, 2, 3.

is found to satisfy (1). Values of z_B and z_C are given in Table 2 for the unknown variance case.

Table 2.

Known Variance Critical Points (Z_B, Z_C) for the Arrow-cross (AC)

Signif.	Corr.	Z_C	Z_B
.05	.50	2.00	3.07
.10	.50	1.71	2.48
.01	.50	2.59	4.65
.05	.40	2.06	2.69

For this Arrow Cross (named for the shape of its no-decision region), (1) is seen to hold for all (θ_1, θ_2) of opposite sign, since then the chance of no misclassification increases with the magnitude of either parameter. For parameters with the same sign, a Neyman-Pearson argument, as in [6], proves that (1) is satisfied as long as $z_C \leq (1+\rho) z_\alpha$, as, for example, with $\rho = .4$ or $.5$ and $\alpha = .05$. For such cases, the AC is the only optimal rule satisfying (1) for all (θ_1, θ_2) values.

How good is the optimal rule? By definition, it is the best rule satisfying (1) when the parameters are near 0. Table 1 indicates that the AC is also good, relative to the rules of [6], when one parameter is near 0. However, when both parameters have the same sign, it does relatively poorly.

6.5. Summary

All four rules considered behave well, none is uniformly best. The only maximin optimal rule satisfying (1) for all (θ_1, θ_2) values is the AC, which is worst when both parameters are equal and away from 0. With this information, the potential user of such rules might well bring other considerations into the choice of a rule. For example, if one wants to be surest of a classification in the case when one of the parameters is near zero, then the AC is probably preferred, while one of the other rules is probably preferred if one is most concerned with performance when both parameters are large.

In brief, the lesson of LaPlace prevails: "Probability is just common sense shored up with a little calculation."

7. The Case of Three Parameters: No Regrets?

For the case of deciding the signs of the three parameters (drugs), a linear program can be defined, analogously to that in Section 6, for determining maximin optimal rules satisfying (1). In this case, the solution is seen to have some of the three-decision regions empty. This says that the best rule when parameters are near 0 can never decide that all parameters have their correct signs, even when the magnitudes of these parameters are arbitrarily large. Surely the rational user would not use the "optimal" rule in such a case.

In this case, the user/statistician has (at least) two options. First, one could seek, from common sense and/or past experience in similar cases, a rule which seems and is verified by some calculations to be reasonable. Such a rule is a Triple Cross extension of the Double Cross.

Alternatively, one could seek a more reasonable optimality criterion and, subsequently, rules which are optimal by this criterion. The trouble with the maximin criterion would seem to be its neglect of what happens when all parameters are not near 0. A way to protect better at such alternatives is to seek to minimize the "regret" of the rule, i.e., the difference between expected correct classifications for this rule and, for example, the rule one would use if the magnitudes, but not the signs, of the parameters were known. And from this point, the author's search for optimal multiple decision rules for the signs of the parameters goes on.

8. Annotated References

[1] Bahadur, R. R. A Property of T-statistics. *Sankhya* 1952-3 12 79-88.

The optimality of [3] for 1 parameter.

[2] Bohrer, Robert. On Bayes Sequential-design with Two Random Variables, *Biometrica 55* (1966), 469-475.

The one optimal lost labels solution.

[3] ____ Multiple Three-decision Rules for Parametric Signs. *J. Am. Statist. Assoc.* (1979) 432-7.

Definition, optimality, and some critical points for the SP Cross.

[4] ____ (with W. Chow, R. Faith, V. M. Joshi, and C.-F. Wu) Multiple Three-decision Rules for Factorial Simple Effects: Bonferroni Wins Again. *J. Am. Statist. Assn.*, 1981 76 119-124.

The geometric probability for SP Cross critical points.

[5] _____ (with Judith Sheft) Misclassification Probabilities in 2^3 Factorial Experiments. *J. Statist. Planning and Inference* (1979) 79-83.

Mathematics underpinning Neyman's 1935 Monte Carlo study to show the need for [3]-[7].

[6] _____ (with Mark Schervish) An Optimal Multiple Decision Rule about Signs. *Proc. Nat. Acad. Sci.* 77 (1980) 52-56.

Derives rules maximizing the minimum expected number of correct decisions subject to a bound on P(no misclassifications).

[7] _____ Our Complements to the 1976 Keynote, to appear in *Statistical Decision Theory and Related Topics, III.* S. S. Gupta, Ed. NY: Academic Press, 1981.

A review of [2]-[6].

[8] Dunnett, C. W. A Multiple Comparisons Procedure for Comparing Several Treatments with a Control *J. Am. Statist. Assn.* 1955 50 1096-1121.

Critical points for a correct solution of the better or no-better problem.

[9] Feldman, D. Contributions to the Two-armed Bandit Problem, *Ann. Math. Statist.* 1962 33 847-856.

The other optimal solution in the missing labels problem.

[10] Kaiser, H. Directional Statistical Decisions, *Psych. Rev.* 1960 67 160-167.

The first step to deciding signs of parameters.

[11] Neyman, J. (with Cooperation of Iwaszkiewicz and Kolodziesczik) Statistical Problems in Agricultural Experimentation, *J. Roy. Statist. Soc. (Suppl.)* 1935 2 107-154.

Introduces goodness criterion for decision rules about signs.

[12] Neyman, J. Discussion of Yates's Paper, *J. Roy. Statist. Soc. (Suppl.)* 1935 2 135-141.

A Monte Carlo study showing the need for [3]-[7].

[13] Spjøtvoll, E. On the Optimality of Some Multiple Comparison Procedures, *Ann. Math. Statist.* 1972 43 398-411.

Motivates use of and essentially proves optimality of the SP Cross in [3], [4], [6].

[14] Tong, Y. L. On Partitioning a Set of Normal Populations. *Ann. Math. Statist.* 1969 40 1300-1324.

Still another sense of optimality, not considered here.

[15] Traxler, R. A Snag in the History of Factorial Experiments in *On the History of Statistics and Probability*. (D. B. Owen, Ed.) NY: Dekker, 1975.

More on Neyman's 1935 Monte Carlo study.

THE LIBRARY
UNIVERSITY OF CALIFORNIA
San Francisco
666-2334

THE BOOK IS DUE ON THE LAST DATE STAMPER BELOW
Books not returned on time are subject to fines according to the Library Lending Code. A renewal may be made on certain materials. For details consult Lending Code.

INTERLIBRARY LOAN
14 DAY
RECEIPT
MAY 5
JUN

Series 4128